Living Dairy-Free

FOR

DUMMIES®

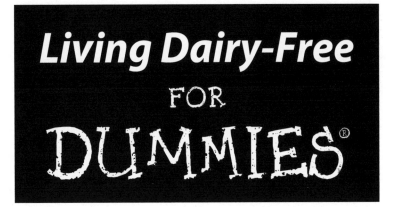

Living Dairy-Free

FOR

DUMMIES®

by Suzanne Havala Hobbs, DrPH

Registered and licensed dietitian

Foreword by John J. B. Anderson, PhD

Emeritus Professor of Nutrition at Gillings School of Global Public Health,
University of North Carolina at Chapel Hill

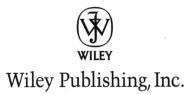

WILEY

Wiley Publishing, Inc.

Living Dairy-Free For Dummies®

Published by
Wiley Publishing, Inc.
111 River St.
Hoboken, NJ 07030-5774
www.wiley.com

Copyright © 2010 by Wiley Publishing, Inc., Indianapolis, Indiana

Published by Wiley Publishing, Inc., Indianapolis, Indiana

Published simultaneously in Canada

For general information on our other products and services, please contact our Customer Care Department within the U.S. at 877-762-2974, outside the U.S. at 317-572-3993, or fax 317-572-4002.

For technical support, please visit www.wiley.com/techsupport.

Wiley also publishes its books in a variety of electronic formats. Some content that appears in print may not be available in electronic books.

Library of Congress Control Number: 2010932437

ISBN: 978-0-470-63316-8

Manufactured in the United States of America

10 9 8 7 6 5 4 3 2 1

WILEY

About the Author

Suzanne Havala Hobbs is a registered, licensed dietitian and nationally recognized writer on food, nutrition, and dietary guidance policy. She holds a doctorate in health policy and administration from the University of North Carolina at Chapel Hill, where she is a clinical associate professor in the Gillings School of Global Public Health — the nation's top public school of public health. There she directs the doctoral program in health leadership and serves on the faculty of the Department of Health Policy and Management and the Department of Nutrition.

An expert on dairy-free living, Sue was the primary author of the American Dietetic Association's 1988 and 1993 position papers on vegetarian diets. She also was the founding chair of the Association's Vegetarian Nutrition Dietetic Practice Group. She serves on the editorial board of *Vegetarian Times* magazine and the advisory boards of the nonprofit Vegetarian Resource Group and the Physicians Committee for Responsible Medicine. She has been living (mostly) dairy-free for 35 years.

Through her popular newspaper column, *On the Table,* Sue explores topics related to food, nutrition, and related policy issues. The column reaches readers weekly through *The News & Observer* of Raleigh, North Carolina, and the discussion continues on her blog at www.onthetable.net.

She has written 12 books, including *Living Vegetarian For Dummies* (Wiley), *Get the Trans Fat Out: 601 Simple Ways to Cut the Trans Fat Out of Any Diet* (Three Rivers Press), *Vegetarian Cooking For Dummies* (Wiley), *The Natural Kitchen: The Complete Guide to Buying and Using Natural Foods and Products* (Berkley), *Good Foods, Bad Foods: What's Left to Eat?* (Wiley), and *Shopping for Health: A Nutritionist's Aisle-by-Aisle Guide to Smart, Low-fat Choices at the Supermarket* (HarperPerennial). She is a contributing writer for *Bottom Line/Personal,* and she also has been a regular writer for *Vegetarian Times, SELF,* and other national publications.

Suzanne is a member of the American Public Health Association, American Dietetic Association, Association of Health Care Journalists, Association of Food Journalists, and the American Society of Journalists and Authors. She served on the board of directors of the Association of Health Care Journalists and the Center for Excellence in Health Care Journalism. She also serves on the board of trustees of the North Carolina Writers' Network.

She lives in Chapel Hill, North Carolina. Her family includes her husband, Michael R. Hobbs, their children, Barbara and Henry, dogs, Kailani and Sperry, and a cat named Kodak.

Dedication

This book is dedicated to people everywhere who strive to eat well to support their health and to protect the well-being of our environment and the other living things with which we share our beautiful planet.

Author's Acknowledgments

Heartfelt thanks to the kind, competent, and hardworking team at Wiley Publishing who made this book possible and expertly guided it from concept to completion: Michael Lewis, Acquisitions Editor; Chad Sievers, Project Editor; Jessica Smith, Copy Editor; and Patrick Redmond, Production Coordinator. I am grateful to Patty Santelli for her assistance with the nutritional analyses of the recipes, and to expert recipe tester Emily Nolan for her good work. I'm especially indebted to my longtime friend and colleague, Reed Mangels, for her help with the technical review. Many thanks go as well to my agents, Mary Ann Naples, formerly of The Creative Culture, as well as to Laura Nolan of DeFiori and Company. It is such a privilege and joy to be part of a team of so many outstanding professionals.

Many of my colleagues in the U.S. and around the world have dedicated their lives and careers to advancing knowledge in nutrition science, the links between diet and health, and the practice of diet and health policymaking. My work builds on theirs, and I salute the collective efforts of this community of scholars and practitioners. I especially thank my colleagues in the Gillings School of Global Public Health at the University of North Carolina at Chapel Hill for their continuing support.

I am grateful for my family and friends and their continued support and good humor. Special thanks to Bob and Laura Bridges and Karen Bush for their hands in helping me juggle writing and skiing in Park City, Utah. My husband, Mike, and my family helped me day-to-day with their encouraging words.

I am indebted, too, to readers of my newspaper column, *On the Table*. Their feedback and encouragement help me stay in touch with issues of primary concern to people trying to do their best to make wise food choices.

Publisher's Acknowledgments

We're proud of this book; please send us your comments at http://dummies.custhelp.com. For other comments, please contact our Customer Care Department within the U.S. at 877-762-2974, outside the U.S. at 317-572-3993, or fax 317-572-4002.

Some of the people who helped bring this book to market include the following:

Acquisitions, Editorial, and Media Development

Senior Project Editor: Chad R. Sievers

Acquisitions Editor: Michael Lewis

Copy Editor: Jessica Smith

Assistant Editor: Erin Calligan Mooney

Senior Editorial Assistant: David Lutton

Technical Editor:
   Reed Mangels, PhD, RD, LDN, FADA

Editorial Manager: Michelle Hacker

Editorial Assistant: Rachelle Amick

Art Coordinator: Alicia B. South

Cover Photos: © iStockphoto.com/parema

Cartoons: Rich Tennant
   (www.the5thwave.com)

Composition Services

Project Coordinator: Patrick Redmond

Layout and Graphics: Samantha K. Cherolis

Illustrator: Elizabeth Kurtzman

Proofreaders: Jessica Kramer, Toni Settle

Indexer: Dakota Indexing

Publishing and Editorial for Consumer Dummies

   Diane Graves Steele, Vice President and Publisher, Consumer Dummies

   Kristin Ferguson-Wagstaffe, Product Development Director, Consumer Dummies

   Ensley Eikenburg, Associate Publisher, Travel

   Kelly Regan, Editorial Director, Travel

Publishing for Technology Dummies

   Andy Cummings, Vice President and Publisher, Dummies Technology/General User

Composition Services

   Debbie Stailey, Director of Composition Services

Contents at a Glance

Recipes at a Glance

Table of Contents

Foreword

*W*henever a major food group is omitted from an individual's diet, it's natural to worry about the potential for nutritional deficiencies. Those concerns may be even greater when the food being removed is such a staple as dairy products. That's especially true for growing children on their way to achieving peak bone mass.

It may surprise you to know, though, that growth records of children raised with no dairy products at all show that they can experience normal and healthy rates of growth. There is, of course, no human requirement for dairy products at all after infancy. And as babies, it's our mother's milk we need, not milk from a cow. Still, to ensure healthy rates of growth and development, the diets of all children — whether or not they drink cow's milk or eat other dairy products — require careful shepherding by their parents.

Good nutrition doesn't just happen. Healthful diets require knowledge and skills. That's where this book comes in. In *Living Dairy-Free For Dummies,* Suzanne Havala Hobbs covers everything you need to know about getting adequate intakes of calcium, vitamin D, and other important nutrients — without eating dairy foods. In addition to adults who want to avoid dairy products, she helps parents plan dairy-free meals that meet the nutritional needs of growing children. Readers will find that the guidelines are laid out clearly in this book, so they are easy to follow.

As a nutrition scientist who has spent decades studying the roles of calcium and vitamin D in human health, I know that nutrition science is complicated, and eating healthfully is not always an easy thing to do in our society. One potential downside of avoiding dairy foods, for example, is evidence that a few nutrients provided in good quantities by milk and other dairy foods may be lower in the diets of people who eat dairy-free diets. This means that alternative food sources of these nutrients need to be eaten.

Calcium and vitamin D are two of the nutrients that need particular attention because of the vital roles they play in bone health. Getting enough calcium and vitamin D to meet recommended levels is no easy feat, whether you eat dairy products or not. With this book as a guide, though, Suzanne Havala Hobbs helps you get what you need.

You don't need dairy products in your diet to be healthy. You do need a quality diet, though, to support your health. For whatever reason you choose to go dairy-free, the practical information in this book will help you get started.

John J. B. Anderson, PhD

Emeritus Professor of Nutrition at the Gillings School of Global Public Health, University of North Carolina at Chapel Hill

Introduction

● ●

*W*hy would anyone think that humans need milk from a cow to be healthy? After all, milk is tailor-made for the species it came from. Dogs drink milk from dog mothers, and giraffes drink milk from giraffe mothers. And cow's milk, for example, is formulated to help calves grow and develop an enormous skeleton in a matter of several months. Human skeletons are small in comparison to cow skeletons, so why would a human need milk that's formulated for fast, enormous bone growth?

Humans are designed to get nourishment from human mothers when they're infants. Human milk contains the nutrients they need in the amounts they need for the growth and development of the *human* body (not the cow body). The milk-drinking phase doesn't last long either — a year to a few years, at most.

In fact, no mammals continue to drink milk after infancy — except humans. And to top it off, the milk that humans drink is from a species other than their own. It's an odd state of affairs, when you think about it. The truth is that humans don't need milk from cows. In fact, they don't need any milk at all once they're grown.

But folks have a strong cultural tradition — perpetuated by powerful political and economic interests, not to mention a love of ice cream — to continue their dairy-filled ways. This tradition causes health problems for some people, because most human adults have at least some level of intolerance to dairy products. This dairy habit also causes unintended environmental and ethical consequences, too. These issues are motivating an increasing number of people to rethink their dairy habits and to live dairy-free. I invite you to use this book to do the same.

About This Book

Living Dairy-Free For Dummies is for anyone with an interest in going dairy-free. It's for folks who may simply want to learn a little more or for those who would like to take the first few steps toward a new, dairy-free lifestyle. Whether you're ready to go part of the way or all the way, this book can help. And no matter the reason you're interested in the dairy-free lifestyle (perhaps your child is allergic to milk, or you're lactose intolerant), you can find the guidance you need here.

Don't feel you need to read the chapters in this book in order from cover to cover. This book is designed to make sense and be helpful whether you surf it casually as you need it or read it in its entirety. Throughout the text, you'll find cross-references to guide you to other parts of the book where you can find related information.

Conventions Used in This Book

To make this book easier to read, the following conventions or rules are followed throughout:

- When introducing a new term that you may not be familiar with, I use *italics* to set it apart. I then follow up with an easy-to-understand definition.
- I **bold** text to highlight keywords in bulleted lists.
- Web addresses are printed in `monofont`. And keep in mind that when this book was printed, some Web addresses may have needed to break across two lines of text. If that happened, rest assured that I haven't put in any extra characters (such as hyphens) to indicate the break. So when using one of these Web addresses, just type in exactly what you see in this book, pretending as though the line break doesn't exist.
- Recipe ingredients aren't specified as being organic, conventional, low-sodium, or any of the other possible variations. When you shop for ingredients, feel free to make these choices as you see fit.
- All temperatures are listed in Fahrenheit.

What You're Not to Read

It's great if you read this entire book from cover to cover. You won't miss any helpful hints and information that way. However, some information I include isn't as critical for you to know. If you need to pare down your reading, here's what you can save for later:

- ✔ **Material flagged with the Technical Stuff icon:** These paragraphs contain information that, while interesting, isn't vital to your understanding of the topic.

- ✔ **Sidebars:** These shaded boxes are scattered throughout the book. The information contained in them is similar to the Technical Stuff: It's great if you have the time, but it isn't critical for you to read.

Foolish Assumptions

If you're holding this book, you or someone who loves you bought or borrowed it to gain a better understanding of how to live a dairy-free lifestyle. This book is appropriate for a variety of purposes, including the following:

- ✔ **Dipping your toe into the topic:** If you just want a little more information to help you decide whether living dairy-free may be something you'd like to consider doing, this book is appropriate for you.

- ✔ **Digging deeper:** You already have a general sense of what's involved in living dairy-free, but you want more in-depth advice about how to do it. If this sounds like your situation, this book is for you.

- ✔ **Sharing the knowledge:** If you know someone with an interest in going dairy-free — or someone who may simply be curious and interested in learning more — this book is a reliable resource.

- ✔ **Refreshing your own knowledge:** People who have been living dairy-free for a long time can benefit from the up-to-date information in this book.

- ✔ **Having a reference on hand:** Health professionals often encounter people with special dietary needs in their work and have to give them medical or dietary advice. If you're a health professional with no personal experience with a dairy-free lifestyle, this book may be helpful as an accurate and quick reference.

You can make some assumptions about me, too:

- ✔ **I know what I'm talking about.** I'm a licensed, registered dietitian with a master's degree in human nutrition and a doctorate in public health. I'm a leading expert on vegetarian diets, which includes variations that exclude all dairy products. Personally, I'm also a vegetarian and have limited my use of dairy products for 35 years.

- ✔ **My advice is practical.** It's informed by my own experience of limiting my intake of dairy products for more than three decades. I also have many years of experience counseling individuals on special diets, including vegetarians, nonvegetarians, and people who avoid dairy products.

✔ **I'm not giving individualized advice.** As much as I wish it were possible, books aren't an appropriate means of dispensing medical or dietary advice tailored to individual needs. I can give you general information that provides a good foundation of knowledge about the topic. However, if you have specific issues you need help with — particularly medical conditions that require you to follow a special diet — you need to get additional, individualized guidance from a registered dietitian. I include information about how to locate a dietitian with expertise in living dairy-free.

How This Book Is Organized

Living Dairy-Free For Dummies is divided into five parts. It's organized to take you through a logical progression of information, moving from basic to more in-depth, depending on your level of interest.

Parts I and II provide fundamental information that you should know if you're contemplating eliminating dairy products from your diet. Parts III and IV are important for anyone ready to dig a little deeper. Part V — the Part of Tens — is downright fun for anyone.

Each part focuses on a different aspect of living dairy-free, including the basic who, what, and why, the ways to get ready to make the transition, the recipes you can try, and the maintenance of the lifestyle over time. Together, the five parts of this book lay the foundation for understanding the dairy-free lifestyle and building the skills necessary to successfully adapt.

Part 1: Going Dairy-Free: A Quick Overview

This part gives a quick summary of the primary areas you need to know as you take steps to go dairy-free. I discuss the basics about what the dairy-free lifestyle is all about: Who may want to go dairy-free and why, nutritional issues, considerations for meal planning, and getting started with the transition.

I dig a little deeper then, and get into more detail about the reasons some people decide to eliminate dairy from their diets. I zero in on lactose intolerance, one of the most common reasons people go dairy-free. I also get into more detail about specific vitamins and minerals you may have questions about and where to get them if you're on a diet without milk. I provide practical pointers about how to steer clear of dairy, including hidden sources and how to find them when you read food labels.

Part II: Setting Up Your Dairy-Free Kitchen

This part explains how to set up a dairy-free kitchen so you can make more meals at home. It covers what you need to know about common and versatile ingredients (and which ones to avoid), where to shop, and strategies for getting the best values. This part also focuses on practical equipment and basic cooking techniques you should know to help you get started.

Part III: Meals Made Easy: Recipes for Everyone

In this part, you can find a good set of starter recipes. The chapters I include address breakfast foods; salads, soups, and sides; main dishes; dips, spreads, sauces, and dressings; breads and munchies; and desserts. The recipes are easy, versatile, and practical. Ingredient lists are short, and basic cooking skills are all that are necessary to follow the simple instructions.

Part IV: Living — and Loving — the Dairy-Free Lifestyle

This part provides in-depth advice for anyone who's ready to take the full plunge into living dairy-free. It includes strategies for preparing meals at home that everyone will love (even those who still eat dairy products) as well as tips for getting along in social situations outside your home, including how to maintain a dairy-free diet when eating at restaurants and when traveling. This part also includes information about going dairy-free at different stages of life, including during pregnancy and infancy, during childhood and as a teen, and throughout your adult years.

Part V: The Part of Tens

Most *For Dummies* books end with The Part of Tens, a collection of handy tips, lists, and fun facts that are easy to read at a glance. This book is no different. The chapters I include in this part provide you with a quick list of reasons to go dairy-free as well as practical advice about how to make it happen, including useful products to try, hidden dairy ingredients to avoid, ways to save money, and ideas for making dairy-free foods fun for kids.

Icons Used in This Book

A fun feature of *For Dummies* books is the inclusion of the clever icons that flag helpful nuggets of information. Each icon denotes a particular type of information. Here's what each type means:

This icon highlights insights or other helpful clues that may make it more convenient or hassle-free for you to follow a dairy-free diet.

When you see this icon, the information that follows is a rule of thumb or another truism you should keep in mind.

If you see this icon, the information is meant to help you avoid a common pitfall or to keep you from getting into trouble.

You'll see this icon attached to information that, while interesting, isn't vital to your understanding of the topic. In other words, some of you may skip it, but it's available if you care to find out more.

Where to Go from Here

The science of nutrition is complicated, but being well nourished is a relatively simple matter. It's even easier to do if you follow good-sense advice about the foods that make up a health-supporting diet. That's where this book comes in.

If you're not sure where to start, peruse the table of contents or index and find a topic that interests you. Otherwise feel free to start at the beginning and read cover to cover.

Whether you go completely dairy-free or just part of the way, using this book as a guide is one of the smartest moves you can make. I hope this book helps. Best wishes to you as you take the first step!

Part I

Going Dairy-Free: A Quick Overview

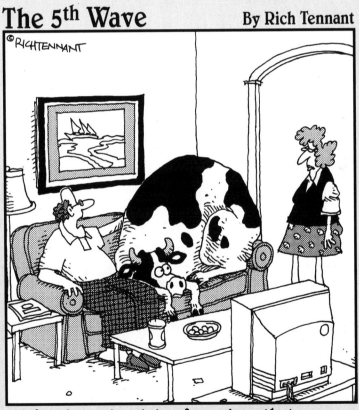

The 5th Wave   By Rich Tennant

"If we're going dairy-free, does that mean you-know-who goes back to the barn?"

In this part . . .

Lifestyle change isn't easy, especially when food is involved. Changing the way you eat requires you to change your mind-set about food. That's the challenge of it, but that's the fun of it, too.

In this part, I introduce you to the basics of living dairy-free. I start with a summary of what dairy-free is all about. I also discuss the health, environmental, and ethical reasons that compel some people to cut dairy products out of their diets. I include a chapter on lactose intolerance — the most common reason people skip bovine beverages and products.

Some of you may be anxious to get answers about the nutrients in dairy products and how to get them on a dairy-free diet. I explain what you need to know in this part.

Finally, I finish up with some practical guidance for avoiding dairy products, including how to stay away from hidden sources of dairy and dairy byproducts and how to spot dairy products on ingredient labels.

Chapter 1

Living Dairy-Free: Beginning with the Basics

....

In This Chapter

▶ Understanding what it means to be dairy-free

▶ Seeing who's avoiding dairy and why

▶ Being well-nourished without milk and dairy products

▶ Planning and preparing satisfying nondairy meals

▶ Making a dairy-free lifestyle work for you

....

*I*f you've picked up this book, you or someone you know may be think-ing about making a major lifestyle change: going dairy-free. It's a big step that may take some getting used to. After all, milk — that bovine beverage that many folks drink with cookies and pour over cereal — is about as all-American as apple pie and corn on the cob. In fact, for most people in North America (and much of Europe, too), milk and foods made from it have been an integral part of everyday life for generations. And tradition is tough to change.

Still, you may be considering doing just that. Why? And how can you make do without a food that was deemed an entire food group in the government's dietary guidelines? I cover these questions and more in this chapter.

In this chapter, I also review what going dairy-free is all about. I explain who may be interested in cutting out dairy and why, discuss how going dairy-free affects your nutritional needs, provide tips for planning and preparing dairy-free meals, and show you how to get started after you've decided to make the switch.

Dairy-Free for You and Me: What It's All About

After infancy, you don't need milk. It's a simple fact. Milk is a substance produced by mammals to nourish their newborn babies. Baby mammals — including humans — depend on milk until their digestive systems have had enough time to mature and allow them to eat solid food. (You can read more about nature's first food and its link to lactose intolerance in Chapter 3.)

After they begin eating solid food, the animals don't go back to drinking milk. That is, of course, unless they're human. Some human adults — a minority of the world's population — drink milk from cows, goats, and other large mammals. Although this practice of milk drinking isn't natural, it goes back to ancient times. Many people like the taste of milk, and it has nutritional value. However, it also has drawbacks — a greater number for some people than for others. The following sections take a closer look the dairy dilemma — why people place importance on milk and why it's a problem for some folks.

Moo juice: Getting the skinny on why milk matters

Milk is a concentrated source of certain nutrients, such as protein, calcium, and the B vitamin riboflavin. Its nutritional value isn't surprising, given that cow's milk is created to help calves grow and develop in a short time into large animals with massive skeletons and musculature. Milk from goats, water buffaloes, and other herd animals is nutritionally similar to cow's milk.

When humans drink milk from one of these large creatures, they get a big dose of protein, vitamins, and minerals in a few gulps. In fact, milk is much more nutritious than many other beverages, including the following:

- **Fruit juice:** This beverage contains no protein or riboflavin. It also contains no calcium, unless it's fortified with the mineral. Depending on the type of juice, it may contain vitamin C, potassium, and other nutrients, though.

- **Soft drinks:** These drinks contain no essential nutrients. They're *empty calorie* drinks, meaning they contain calories but have no nutritional value in exchange for those calories. In other words, soft drinks are junk.

- **Coffee, tea, and water:** These beverages are in a different category. They contain no calories or essential nutrients (unless you add sugar and creamer, of course). They're simply fluids, and generally they're beneficial because they hydrate you. Caffeinated drinks, such as coffee and tea, contain substances that cause you to lose some fluid, but you gain far more fluid than you lose.

As compared with other beverages, milk is nutritious. That doesn't mean you need it, though. And along with the benefits, drinking cow's milk has some significant drawbacks. Depending on the type of milk or dairy products you eat, some dairy foods may be better or worse for you than others. As a matter of fact, some people can't drink milk at all. Why? Keep reading.

Understanding when a "good thing" is the wrong thing

Sure, drinking milk has its benefits (see the preceding section), but as soon as you were eating apples and oatmeal as a child, you didn't need your mother's milk any more. You certainly didn't need milk from a cow when you were a baby, and that hasn't changed in adulthood.

In fact, most people lose their ability to digest milk. If they drink milk or eat dairy products, these folks experience a variety of unpleasant symptoms. Those symptoms, which may range from bloating and abdominal pain to cramps and diarrhea, are signs that their bodies are no longer equipped to handle milk. I cover this issue of lactose intolerance in detail in Chapter 3. In the long term, including milk in your diet may affect you in other ways, too, regardless of whether you can digest milk. (See the later section "Why do you do it? Looking at the many reasons for living dairy-free.")

Being a dairy detective

Dairy products are widespread, so if you're considering going dairy-free, you need to be aware of where dairy rears its ugly head in everyday foods. Doing without dairy requires being conscious of the varied places milk and milk products are used.

You easily can find the obvious sources of milk, including a glass of milk served with a slice of chocolate cake or the milk used to make pudding, ice cream, or cream of broccoli soup. Milk also is used to make yogurt, whipped cream, cream cheese, and other cheeses.

But even if you don't see them, dairy products are used in many other foods as well. Byproducts of milk, such as skim milk solids and casein, sometimes are used as ingredients in processed foods, including commercial piecrust, cookies, and crackers.

Small bits of dairy may be used in foods when you eat out, too. For example, Parmesan cheese often is added to Caesar salads, and buttermilk may be used to make a stack of pancakes. I include more examples of places you'll find dairy — including hidden sources of dairy ingredients — in Chapters 5 and 22.

Doing without Dairy: Who Is Affected and Why

Like me, you may have been raised in a family or community where drinking milk and eating dairy products was the norm. You enjoyed drinking milk-shakes and eating ice cream with your friends, and you ate grilled cheese sandwiches with your cream of tomato soup. You likely dunked your cookies into a glass of cold milk as well. And, of course, you kept a gallon of milk in your refrigerator at all times.

But you also may have known someone who didn't drink milk. That person may have said that she didn't like the taste of milk. Another common explanation is, "I like milk, but it doesn't like me." Today, it's much more common to meet people who don't eat dairy products, and that number is increasing rapidly. The following sections take a closer look at the people who live dairy-free and why they do so.

Getting a snapshot of who's going dairy-free

In some countries, dairy foods aren't a major component of the culture's diet. In fact, they may not be eaten at all. In parts of Asia, for example, soymilk is much more common than cow's milk. In India, milk is used to make cheese, pudding, and yogurt, but these foods are eaten in small quantities as condiments or occasional treats. In Africa, some people don't drink any form of milk at all.

As more people from other countries move to the United States, they bring with them their food traditions. They open restaurants and ethnic grocery stores and sell foods from their native countries. These newcomers also are a growing market for products such as the soymilk, almond milk, and nondairy cheeses you may have noticed showing up more frequently in your neighbor-hood supermarket.

All this mobility around the world is creating a shift in eating habits and driving more people to go dairy-free. Newcomers to dairy-centric parts of the world, such as the United States and Canada, may already be used to a diet that's largely dairy-free. And they're exposing everybody else to the alternatives to the preferred dairy products. When given the choice, you may opt to go dairy-free. If that's the case, it's easier than ever to do.

Why do you do it? Looking at the many reasons for living dairy-free

Going dairy-free makes a lot of sense for your health and for the environment. And, of course, different people do it for different reasons. Among those reasons are the following:

- ✔ **They can't digest cow's milk.** Most of the world's adults can't completely digest cow's milk. Some have so much difficulty digesting milk that they develop unpleasant symptoms, such as gas, bloating, abdominal cramps, and diarrhea, when they drink milk or eat other dairy products.

- ✔ **They want to support the health of the planet.** Animal agriculture, including the production and distribution of milk and other dairy products, takes a toll on the earth. It contributes to air and water pollution and global warming. It also requires large amounts of fossil fuels and fresh water supplies, and it plays a part in the overuse of antibiotics.

- ✔ **They have compassion for animals and people.** Modern methods of dairy farming raise ethical concerns about the manner in which animals are treated on factory farms. The dairy industry is associated with the meat industry, where retired dairy cows join animals raised for their meat. The animals are processed in slaughterhouses where animals are treated inhumanely and conditions are dangerous for workers.

- ✔ **They just don't like the taste of milk.** They may not find the taste or texture appealing, or they may be turned off by the thought of drinking mammary secretions from cows.

- ✔ **They want to take better care of their health.** Although dairy products do have some benefits, you can like dairy too much. It can be detrimental to your health in the amounts that Americans typically consume it. See the nearby sidebar "Contemplating the enormous amounts of dairy products in the standard American diet" to consider how much dairy the average person consumes.

Milk is devoid of dietary fiber, and it's high in artery-clogging saturated fat. When you drink milk or eat dairy products regularly, you risk pushing out of your diet foods you need in greater quantities, such as vegetables, fruits, and whole grains. You also raise your blood cholesterol levels and increase your risk for coronary artery disease, which can lead to a heart attack or stroke.

Generally, all these dairy-free folks like the convenience of alternatives such as soymilk, rice milk, and almond milk that are on the market now. I discuss the health, environmental, and ethical rationales for going dairy-free in greater detail in Chapters 2 and 20.

Contemplating the enormous amounts of dairy products in the standard American diet

In countries like the United States and Canada, milk and other milk products play a prominent role in meals. If you're like a lot of people, you may melt cheese over your broccoli and tortilla chips. You also may add it to sandwiches, pizza, and casseroles. And you may eat chunks of cheese on crackers. You may even bread your favorite cheese and deep-fry it as an appetizer.

And if that's not enough, think about milk sold in gallon jugs. You pour it on your cereal in the morning and drink it as a beverage with meals. You may eat yogurt and ice cream and cream cheese on bagels and in cheesecake, and you may top potatoes, burritos, and ice cream sundaes and other desserts with sour cream and whipped cream. You may eat huge quantities of dairy products. It's too much for your body to handle.

Getting the Nutrients You Need

If you were raised in a milk-centric culture, you probably equate drinking cow's milk with having strong bones and teeth. It's natural then to wonder — or even worry — about how you'll get what your body needs if you don't drink milk or eat other dairy products. The good news is that you don't need dairy products to get the nutrients you need.

Any health-supporting diet takes care and planning, whether or not it includes dairy products. Still, it's reassuring to know that there's no requirement for you to drink milk to be healthy. This section may put your milk concerns at ease.

If you don't drink milk or consume other dairy products, where do you get your calcium, vitamin D, riboflavin, and other nutrients typically associated with these products? It's one of the first questions your friends and family will ask you if you tell them you're going dairy-free. Rest assured that these nutrients are widely available in many other health-supporting foods. You probably already enjoy some of them.

You can find calcium in navy bean soup, almonds, fortified orange juice, and cooked kale. Sunshine is nature's natural source of vitamin D, though you also can get it in eggs and certain kinds of fish. Riboflavin and other vitamins, as well as all the minerals and other substances you need for good health, are widespread in other foods, too, including a range of fruits, vegetables, beans and peas, seeds, nuts, and whole grains. These are the healthiest foods you can possibly eat. (I delve deeper into these nutrients in Chapter 4.)

You can find plenty of nutrients in foods that may be new to you, too. If you don't mind experimenting a bit, some of these products may become new favorites. Examples include soymilk, almond milk, rice milk, nondairy cheese, soy yogurt, and other nondairy products. Most of them taste great and work in recipes in much the same way that cow's milk and traditional dairy products do. I discuss your nondairy food choices, including where to find the products and how to select them, in Chapters 6 and 7.

Digging In to Dairy-Free Meal Planning and Preparation

Before you can go dairy-free, you need to soak up some knowledge and master a few new skills. Among the most important things you need to get a handle on are planning and preparing nutritious, good-tasting meals.

The more foods you fix for yourself at home, the more control you have over your diet. By preparing foods from scratch, you can more easily monitor the ingredients used and ensure that your meals are dairy-free.

The following sections give you the lowdown on removing the dairy from your kitchen, shopping for the products you need, and beginning to whip up some tasty dairy-free recipes at home.

Preparing to de-dairy your kitchen

To fix your own dairy-free meals, you need to have the right ingredients on hand. But before you stock up on staples, you must purge your refrigerator and pantry of milk, milk products, and any packaged or processed foods made with dairy ingredients.

Look for and get rid of milk, cheese, yogurt, and ice cream. Remove margarine, sour cream, whipped cream, and cream cheese, too. Read food labels to check for hidden sources of dairy. Give away these unwanted dairy products to friends and family members outside your home. Or throw away amounts that are too small to keep.

The point is to remove these foods from sight so they don't distract you or create a psychological barrier to change. Leaving dairy products in your kitchen may make it too easy to fall back into old patterns of cooking and eating. Be thorough. I share more advice about ways to rid your home and your diet of dairy products in Chapters 5 and 6. After the dairy products are banished, you're ready to bring in the replacements, which I discuss in the next section.

Selecting dairy-free supplies

Before you head to the store for your dairy-free supplies, sit down and think about what you need. Doing so increases your likelihood of having all the necessary staples to make a variety of appealing meals at home. Planning ahead also makes it more likely that you won't forget to pick up a key ingredient, saving you the time and hassle of a return trip to the store.

In between shopping trips, keep a running list of foods you need. A slip of paper attached to the refrigerator or cupboard door or on a notepad at the kitchen desk is a great way to keep a grocery list. Just don't forget to take it with you when you leave for the store. Or you can create a working list in your cellphone or PDA, which you probably carry with you at all times. Then, when you're at the store, you can pull out your phone and voilà, you have your list.

Where you shop is up to you, but many good, dairy-free products are available in more stores than ever before. Natural foods stores carry the widest range of nondairy products, such as soymilk, rice milk, almond milk, soy yogurt, nondairy cheese, and others. Because dairy-free foods are gaining in popularity, your regular neighborhood supermarket also is likely to carry some of these products. If you don't see what you want, ask the store manager about placing a special order.

As you think about the foods you want to buy, keep these pointers in mind:

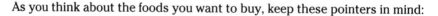

- ✔ **Comparison shop.** Private-label and store brands of popular, nondairy staples, such as soymilk, rice milk, and nondairy coffee creamer, may be high in quality but significantly cheaper than name brands. These products often are a good value. Prices of the same products can vary among stores, too, so shop around.

- ✔ **Buy for versatility.** If you buy plain soymilk or plain nondairy yogurt instead of sweetened, flavored varieties, you can use them in recipes that are sweet or savory.

    For example, plain soymilk or rice milk can be poured over your cereal at breakfast, but it also can be used to make mashed potatoes for dinner. Vanilla-flavored milk, on the other hand, may taste great on cereal, but it wouldn't be a good choice in mashed potatoes or a quiche.

- ✔ **Read food labels carefully.** Scour ingredient labels to be sure the products you're buying are dairy-free. Small amounts of added dairy ingredients may be hidden in products you wouldn't suspect. I include lists of hidden dairy ingredients in Chapters 5 and 22.

To read more strategies for shopping and filling your home with nondairy staples, check out Chapter 7.

Cooking dairy-free

Adapting your cooking style to accommodate dairy-free meals is relatively easy. That's because most nondairy substitutes for common dairy products behave similarly in recipes. For example, you can use nondairy milks — soy, almond, rice, and others — cup for cup in place of cow's milk in any recipe. You also can use dairy-free cheeses in many of the same ways that you always used dairy-based cheeses.

A few caveats are in order, but they aren't difficult to accommodate. For instance, some nondairy forms of cheese don't melt as well as dairy-based varieties. The fix? Mix the nondairy cheese into a hot, moist dish, such as a bowl of pasta or a casserole. The heat and moisture help the cheese to melt more completely.

I cover the ins and outs of cooking using nondairy ingredients in more detail in Chapter 8. For the most part, though, nondairy counterparts to traditional, dairy-based ingredients are easy to work with and taste great. They make it possible to continue to enjoy macaroni and cheese, cheesy nachos, or a glass of milk with your cookies — all dairy-free.

In addition to using these nondairy products, the other aspect of cooking dairy-free is simply exploring and adopting a greater range of foods in your diet that happen to be dairy-free. Consider the following examples:

- ✔ Many people find that pizza made with a variety of tasty toppings — minus the cheese — is a delicious and more healthful alternative to the gooey, greasy, cheesy varieties you may have eaten in the past.

- ✔ Whole-wheat pasta tossed with olive oil, basil, freshly steamed vegetables, toasted pine nuts, and chopped, fresh tomatoes — minus the cheese — is a sophisticated and satisfying alternative to dishes that are coated with salty commercial tomato sauce and gobs of melted cheese.

I provide plenty more examples of the foods you can experiment with in Part III. In this part, you can find dozens of quick and easy recipes to help you get started.

Moving toward a Dairy-Free Lifestyle

Making diet changes is challenging for most people. You not only need to educate yourself about the lifestyle change and master new skills, but you also have to change your mindset about the way you eat. These tasks take time, patience, and work.

It also helps to have support from the people around you, including your family, friends, and co-workers. Throughout this book, I help you think about ways to recruit that support from those around you and how to minimize distractions that may otherwise threaten to derail your best efforts. Part IV is a great place to start. In that part, I cover how to respond in social settings and when away from home as you're incorporating a dairy-free lifestyle. I also discuss dairy-free living throughout the many stages of life. I get you started in the following sections.

Dealing with food in your relationships

Whether it's the people closest to you — your immediate family and best friends — or those you work with at the office or in the community, food usually plays an important role in your relationships. Food traditions help people bond with one another. They bring people together and provide a common experience that most people value in their lives. Consider, for example, the happy memories you have of holiday meals or potluck dinners with your family and friends.

However, when you have a diet restriction that distinguishes you from others in your life, you may experience some tension in those relationships. So, it's a good idea to do what you can to bridge the differences and minimize the extent to which your dairy-free diet may prevent you from fully sharing or participating in meals with others.

You can minimize the extent to which your dairy-free diet affects your relationships in a number of ways. Maintaining a positive attitude and staying as flexible as possible are two good ways to help. Good examples of this advice in action include the following:

- ✔ **Asking for input:** Among your family members, discuss dairy-free meal options and ask for opinions about what everybody would like to eat. Make a list of nondairy dishes that everyone likes and make those dishes often.

    Giving family members a voice and a vote on what you serve at meals is important. People who participate in meal planning are more likely to feel a sense of buy-in and be more satisfied with the outcome as a result.

- ✔ **Compromising with solutions:** Discuss compromises to make meal planning less work. For example, instead of making two different entrees — one with cheese and one without — brainstorm options that keep you from having double the work.

    For example, you may opt to make a dairy-free pasta tossed with garlic, olive oil, and vegetables one night for everyone at the table — dairy eaters and those who avoid dairy alike. At the next meal, you may opt to serve a dairy-loaded entree and a salad. You can allow the salad to pull double duty as a side dish for dairy eaters and an entree salad for others. Add garbanzo beans and sunflower seeds for protein and crunch.

I provide some more detailed examples of how to make meal planning in a mixed household (some dairy eaters and some avoiders) easier in Chapter 15. Going dairy-free with your children can be particularly challenging, but it is doable. Check out Chapter 18 for loads of child-friendly tips and strategies.

Managing your diet outside the home

Just as developing skills for dealing with diet differences inside your home is important, understanding how to manage relationships when you're away is essential. You can anticipate situations in which you'll be a guest at somebody's home for dinner and think about the most comfortable way to broach the topic of your food preferences with your host.

For example, should you tell your host at the time of the invitation? Should you offer to bring a dish? Or would you rather keep your diet difference to yourself, take your chances, and dodge the dairy as necessary? The choice is yours, but it's one you should give some thought to before being faced with the dilemma. Thinking about the possibility ahead of time makes the decision clearer to you the next time you're faced with the situation.

Of course, you'll eat out at places other than people's homes, too — at restaurants, for example. So you'll need a set of skills for sticking to your dairy-free diet at the many different types of eating establishments. Some restaurants are more likely than others to provide you with a range of appropriate dairy-free menu choices. Many ethnic restaurants, including those that serve Chinese, Ethiopian, and Middle Eastern foods, traditionally include a good number of menu items made without milk or cheese.

If you're unsure about the menu, be assertive and ask your server questions about how foods are prepared. Better restaurants will make your food to order, giving you the option to omit the dairy. I cover these issues related to eating away from home in more detail in Chapters 15 and 16.

Experiencing a dairy-free lifestyle during all of life's stages

Living dairy-free is a fine choice throughout your entire life. After early infancy (when, technically, no one is dairy-free), children, teens, and adults of all ages can safely live without milk. I describe dietary considerations for all these times of your life in Chapters 17, 18, and 19.

A good diet is one that supports health for the long term. It's an eating style you can stick with — and enjoy — forever. Living dairy-free can meet both of these goals. Unlike fad diets that ask you to eat nothing but cabbage soup or cookies for weeks on end, living dairy-free is natural. Humans don't require cow's milk, so avoiding milk and dairy products isn't harmful in any way. On the contrary, for many people, continuing to eat dairy foods compromises their health. For whatever reason you choose to go dairy-free, do it with confidence.

Chapter 2

Understanding Why Living Dairy-Free Makes Sense

For many people, eating dairy products is a way of life. Maybe it is for you, too. If so, you may find it difficult to imagine life without an ice cream cone, cookies and milk, or a heaping plate of macaroni and cheese. You may not know how to cook custard or quiche without milk or cream. And you may wonder, "What's a baked potato without sour cream?" At some point, though, many people find that for a variety of reasons eating dairy products is the wrong choice for their lifestyle.

The most common reason people consider going dairy-free is for their health. A number of health issues are related to eating dairy products. In this chapter, I introduce each one and summarize the reasons they make sense — or don't. Beyond health, I discuss another important reason that motivates some people to go dairy-free: the environment. Some compelling reasons exist why eating fewer dairy products may have a role in protecting the quality of the earth's soil, water, and air. Finally, I cover the ethical issues surrounding the impact of the human dairy habit on cows as well as the potent economic and political forces that keep dairy foods on people's plates.

For the Health of It: Avoiding Negative Health Effects of Dairy Products

As a human, you share a common place in the animal kingdom along with other primates, such as monkeys, chimps, and gorillas. You're an *omnivore,* which means you can get along for a short time eating just about anything you want.

In the long run, though, the optimal diet for all humans — the diet that keeps humans the healthiest, the longest — is made primarily of plants. That means your body performs best when you eat foods that come from the soil, such as fruits, vegetables, grains, legumes, seeds, and nuts.

When you were a baby, you were dependent on your mother to feed you. The perfect food, customized just for you, was your human mother's milk. After you were old enough to begin eating solid food from your family's table, your body stopped needing your mother's milk, and you made the transition to toddlerhood and beyond. "Beyond" is the point where milk gets many people into trouble.

Most adult humans aren't designed to continue consuming milk after infancy. That's true of human milk, and it's especially true of cow's milk. In this section, I explain how a milk habit can affect your health and why you may want to consider going dairy-free.

Health effect #1: Many adults are lactose intolerant

While you're a baby, your body produces an enzyme called *lactase* that enables you to digest *lactose,* the natural sugar in milk. Milk tastes pretty good, and it provides you with what you need to grow and develop when you're an infant. As you grow into childhood, though, your body gradually stops making lactase. At this time, babies begin eating baby rice cereal and begin reaching for the crackers in their parents' hands. By the time most people are adults, they don't produce much, if any, lactase. They also don't drink milk — or at least that's what's supposed to happen.

Passing undigested milk sugar into your intestines may cause you to develop symptoms when you eat dairy products. It may cause gastrointestinal problems such as gas, bloating, nausea, abdominal cramps, and diarrhea. When these symptoms appear, the condition is known as *lactose intolerance.* Its cause is a normal condition, and it's one of the major reasons that many people prefer to avoid dairy products.

For reasons I cover in Chapter 3, a small proportion of the world's adult population can actually digest cow's milk pretty well. They can continue drinking milkshakes and eating cheese on their pizza with no immediate concerns. The majority of people, though, have some level of lactose malabsorption.

Health effect #2: Some people suffer from milk allergies

Some people confuse lactose malabsorption or intolerance with milk allergy. But, in reality, they're two completely different health issues. Lactose intolerance, as noted in the preceding section, is caused by the body's inability to digest the milk sugar lactose.

A milk allergy, on the other hand, is an extreme response by the body's immune system to proteins in milk. Cow's milk has many different proteins. Casein is one example; it's the protein that's often used as an ingredient in processed foods. (I include examples of those foods in Chapter 5.) Milk allergy reactions can include hives, rashes, nausea, congestion, diarrhea, swelling in the mouth and throat, and other symptoms. Severe reactions can even lead to shock and death.

About 2.5 percent of children under the age of 3 have milk allergies, according to the American Academy of Allergy, Asthma, & Immunology. The allergy usually shows up in the first year of life. The good news is that 80 percent of children with a milk allergy outgrow it by the time they're 16 years old.

Goat's milk isn't a safe substitute for cow's milk for someone with a milk allergy. Goat's milk is too similar in composition to cow's milk. If someone is allergic to the proteins in cow's milk, she'll likely be allergic to the protein in goat's milk, too.

Managing milk allergies

A milk allergy — like all food allergies — can be tricky to manage. That's because you'll encounter some special challenges when trying to avoid milk proteins. These challenges include the following:

- ✔ **The presence of hidden milk proteins:** As I discuss in Chapter 5, the milk protein casein can turn up in processed foods, restaurant foods, and foods you may eat at someone's home. Because these foods don't always come with detailed ingredient lists, you may find it difficult to know for certain what they contain.

  The key to successfully avoiding milk protein in these cases is to be assertive and ask for information about what's in the food. If the wait staff or your hosts don't know, ask to see package labels of foods you suspect may contain casein. In Chapters 15 and 16, I provide more information on managing social situations and dodging dairy when eating out.

- ✔ **Cross-contamination:** Milk residues that contain protein may inadvertently end up in other foods. For example, a spoon used to mix a bowl of pudding (made with milk) may be used to stir a pot of oatmeal, adding a trace of milk protein to the oatmeal. This cross-contamination also can take place during manufacturing. However, food labels are required to note when foods are prepared on shared equipment and cross contamination with an allergen is a risk.

A trace may be all it takes to set off an allergic reaction. Individuals' sensitivities to food allergens vary. Depending on a person's level of sensitivity, it may take more or less of an allergen to trigger a reaction.

Protecting yourself or your loved one

Handling a milk allergy requires vigilance. To protect yourself or your loved one, you should follow this basic advice:

✔ **Be ready.** Heed your healthcare provider's advice about how to be prepared for emergencies. In some cases, you may want to have injectable epinephrine and antihistamines handy at all times.

✔ **Take no chances.** Be assertive and ask about ingredients in food when you or your allergic family member is eating away from home.

✔ **Read food labels carefully.** Be aware of foods that may harbor small amounts of milk protein. I list examples in Chapter 5.

Two good resources for more information about milk allergies include

✔ The Food Allergy & Anaphylaxis Network, or FAAN (www.food allergy.org/page/milk-allergy)

✔ The American Academy of Allergy, Asthma, & Immunology (www.aaaai.org)

Health effect #3: A dairy-heavy diet may hurt your heart health

Heart disease is the leading killer of both men and women, so it makes a whole lot of sense to do what you can to minimize your risk. Although you can't eliminate all risk factors in life — such as your genetic background — you can focus on what you do have power to control. Your lifestyle is a major factor in determining heart health, and diet is an important component of that. That's where dairy comes in.

Along with red meats, dairy products are the biggest source of *saturated fat* in most Americans' diets. Saturated fats stimulate your body to produce more *cholesterol*. Cholesterol is a waxy substance found in the hard plaques inside diseased arteries. Those plaques cause a narrowing of the arteries to the heart (or the brain), setting you up for a variety of health risks, including heart attack and stroke. This condition is referred to as *coronary artery disease*.

Autism is speculated to be linked to casein consumption

Autism is a developmental disorder that affects an individual's social and communication skills and often includes repetitive behaviors. It usually becomes apparent in early childhood, and it lasts a lifetime. A cure for autism doesn't yet exist, but many researchers are trying to uncover clues to better understand the causes and potential treatments or cures. Dietary factors are among the angles being studied, including the relationship between autism and the milk protein casein (as well as *gluten*, a wheat protein).

Though some advocacy groups have recommended a gluten-free, casein-free diet to treat autism, the science doesn't currently support this approach as having any effect on the condition. A casein-free diet isn't likely to cause any harm, but it doesn't appear to have any benefit either. As a result, more research is needed before doctors and experts recommend a casein-free diet to treat autism.

For people with a predisposition to developing this disease, high blood cholesterol levels are associated with a greater risk. In fact, the Institute of Medicine of the National Academies has reported that no safe intake level of saturated fat exists. In general, the greater your intake of saturated fat, the greater your risk of clogged arteries.

About two-thirds of the fat in dairy products is artery-clogging saturated fat. In particular, hard cheeses (such as cheddar, Swiss, and provolone), ice cream, sour cream, whipped cream, coffee cream, and whole milk are exceptionally high in saturated fat. Premium brands of ice cream are, in general, loaded with saturated fat. Eat them seldom — or never.

Even so-called low-fat dairy products are high in saturated fat. For example, low-fat or 2-percent milk gets 25 percent of its calories from fat, most of which is saturated fat. That's too much saturated fat for most people. Skim or ½-percent milk are the only forms of cow's milk recommended in general for people who drink it, including everyone older than 1 year of age.

The only way to avoid getting too much saturated fat from dairy products is to choose only nonfat varieties or to use dairy products like cheese and sour cream sparingly — like a condiment. Or, even better, just go dairy-free. Avoiding dairy products is a good way of reducing your risk of coronary artery disease and stroke.

Health effect #4: Dairy products can exacerbate certain health issues

Some people choose to avoid dairy products to improve their health even though a proven cause-and-effect relationship doesn't necessarily exist between their condition and the consumption of dairy products.

Basically, these folks suspect that dairy products simply may be related to their problem. If they eliminate dairy and their condition improves — great! They have nothing to lose by trying, because humans just don't require milk from a cow. The following sections identify a few health issues that can potentially improve by going dairy-free.

Irritable bowel syndrome (IBS)

Irritable bowel syndrome (IBS) is one example of a health issue people have that may be alleviated by going dairy-free. IBS is a catchall term that refers to bowel disorders that share a collection of symptoms for which there's no known cause.

Some of the symptoms of IBS may be similar to those of lactose intolerance, including chronic abdominal pain and bloating. IBS often includes changes in bowel movements that may range from constipation to diarrhea.

So, when experimenting with ways to alleviate the symptoms of IBS, some people eliminate dairy products. Considering the high prevalence of lactose malabsorption in adults around the world, it's certainly possible that going dairy-free may help some people.

Ovarian cancer

Some scientists are pursuing research examining a potential link between high intakes of lactose — the amount found in three cups of milk per day — and increased risk of ovarian cancer. More research is needed before conclusions can be drawn. However, an analysis of 500,000 women found that those with high intakes of lactose had higher risks of ovarian cancer when compared to women with lower lactose intakes. The scientists found no association between overall intakes of milk or dairy products and risk of ovarian cancer, however.

One theory as to how the lactose-ovarian cancer connection may work pertains to the role of a byproduct of lactose digestion. When lactose is digested, it's broken down into a smaller sugar, *galactose.* Some scientists believe that high levels of galactose may damage the ovaries and lead to ovarian cancer. Other researchers have suggested that processing cow's milk at dairy plants may alter the hormones in milk in a way that increases the risk of ovarian and other hormone-related cancers.

Tackling special considerations for babies and new moms

The topic of milk takes on special significance for babies and their mothers. The best food for human babies is human breast milk. It's specially designed to deliver precisely the right nutrients in the right amounts for optimal infant growth and development. Breastfeeding also offers health benefits to a new mom, because it helps her uterus contract and return to its pre-pregnancy state. It also helps her lose excess "baby weight." In fact, a woman who breastfeeds her baby burns 500 calories a day more than when she isn't breastfeeding. A deficit of 500 calories a day adds up to a weight loss of about one pound per week.

Sometimes, though, it's not possible for a woman to breastfeed her baby. In those cases, the mother's milk has to be replaced with baby formula, a synthetic substitute designed to be as nutritionally similar to human milk as possible. Some baby formulas are made with a soy base, and others are made with a cow's milk base. Problems can come up when a baby is allergic to either cow's milk or soy. I discuss this in more detail in Chapter 17.

Pregnancy and breastfeeding also are times when a woman has higher nutritional needs to support her and her baby's health. She has less room in her diet for junky, low-nutrition foods and a greater need for a wide range of vitamins, minerals, protein, fats, and carbohydrates. Cow's milk is a rich source of many of these nutrients, so is it okay for a pregnant woman or new mom to avoid consuming it? Yep. Many other foods contain the same nutrients. It bears repeating: Humans don't need milk from a cow. I cover the nutritional ins and outs of eating a dairy-free diet in Chapter 4, and I focus specifically on dairy-free nutrition during pregnancy and infancy in Chapter 17.

Prostate cancer

Research suggests a link between milk consumption and increased risk for prostate cancer. A Harvard study of male health professionals who drank two or more glasses of milk per day yielded findings that suggest relatively high intakes of milk and/or calcium may be related to higher risks of advanced or fatal cases of prostate cancer. Going dairy-free may reduce this risk.

Health effect #5: Eating dairy can promote weight gain

The million-dollar question these days seems to be, "Can drinking milk help you lose weight?" The short answer: No. In recent years, the dairy industry has promoted a marketing campaign touting the weight-loss benefits of drinking cow's milk. Claims that suggest drinking milk controls weight are misleading.

Long-term studies show no benefits for weight loss by drinking cow's milk or eating yogurt.

If anything, drinking lots of milk would be expected to promote weight gain in the long run. That's because fluid cow's milk is relatively high in calories, especially if it's low-fat or whole milk instead of skim. Research on the relationship between beverage consumption and weight control suggests that most people don't compensate for calories consumed from beverages. For example, if they drink a 200-calorie glass of milk, they don't necessarily compensate by eating 200 fewer calories elsewhere in their diets. In other words, people who drink caloric beverages consume those calories on top of the calories from everything else they consume during the day. So, controlling your weight by drinking milk is a tactic that's likely to work poorly.

High-fat dairy products, such as cheese and ice cream, also are high in calories. Just like fluid cow's milk, they promote weight gain and obesity when eaten frequently or in large amounts as is customary in the United States, Canada, and parts of Europe.

Saving the Planet with Your Knife and Fork

Some people go dairy-free because of health reasons (see the earlier section "For the Health of It: Avoiding Negative Health Effects of Dairy Products" for details). Others give it up because they just don't like milk. They don't like the flavor, or maybe they find the notion that they're drinking a bovine bodily fluid unappealing. I know at least one person who gave up all dairy products after eating a serving of cottage cheese that had spoiled.

And, finally, other people are acutely aware of the links between what they eat and the health of the planet. Just as aesthetics may motivate some people to avoid dairy, the thought of how the dairy industry affects the environment compels others to act. They avoid dairy products as a way of making an individual contribution to preserving the environment and the quality of the planet's soil, water, and air. In this section, I share details about the link between dairy products and environmental concerns. See whether any of these issues speak to you.

Contemplating climate change

Abundant evidence shows that mass animal agriculture — the meat and dairy industries — contribute substantially to the production of the gases believed to cause climate change. Climate change is a growing concern around the world. In the coming years, changes in the planet's climate brought on, in part, by humanity's dependence on animal foods, are projected to cause shortages of food, water, and arable land in various parts of the world.

Even if these shortages happen "over there," everyone will be affected. Food and water shortages cause political instability and can affect availability or costs of food supplies everywhere. Because everyone is connected in the global economy, everyone also is affected by each other's misfortunes. You can make an individual contribution to solving the problem of climate change by what you choose to eat — or not eat.

The U.N. Food and Agriculture Organization in 2006 reported that livestock production for meat and milk accounts for about one-fifth of the world's greenhouse gas production. That's more than the greenhouse gases produced by all the world's cars, trucks, planes, trains, and boats put together. For a comprehensive look at the roles of meat and dairy products in climate change, read the report, "Livestock's Long Shadow," available online from the U.N. Food and Agriculture Organization at www.fao.org/docrep/010/a0701e/a0701e00.HTM. Also see the United Nations Environment Programme site at www.unep.org/climatechange.

For more information about how to cut down on your meat intake, see my book *Living Vegetarian For Dummies* (Wiley).

Conserving and protecting the soil, water, and air

Steps for delaying or halting climate change involve protecting the planet's natural resources, including the soil, water, and air. Some of the ways the production and distribution of meat and milk products affect the environment include

✔ **Deforestation:** Huge areas of the earth's landmass are used for cattle grazing. With fewer trees, less carbon dioxide is absorbed from the atmosphere. And more carbon dioxide is released when trees are burned to clear grazing land.

✔ **Noxious emissions:** Animals raised for meat and milk produce manure that sends nitrous oxide into the atmosphere. *Nitrous oxide* is a gas with nearly 300 times the warming power of carbon dioxide. It isn't the only gas that animals produce either. Cows pass gas, too — lots of it. The methane they produce has a more powerful warming effect than carbon dioxide.

✔ **Intensive use of resources:** Meat and milk production and distribution require the use of fossil fuels and huge quantities of water. Industrial feedlots drain water supplies and also pollute the air, water, and soil. Consider the following:

- Petroleum, a fossil fuel, is used for transporting animals and their feed far distances. It's also used for running farm machinery and operating factory farms.

- Pesticides, herbicides, and fertilizers used to raise animals for meat and milk products get washed into streams, rivers, lakes, and bays and contaminate the water supply. Ditto for the nitrogen-containing feces produced by these animals. Because of this pollution, less clean water is available for people, and the creatures that live in these fresh bodies of water are dying off, too.

Because of these effects, some people choose their foods not only by their nutritional value but also by their environmental score. Of course, going dairy-free would garner a low (favorable) environmental score (and also may offer health advantages).

The Swedish government is testing new food labels that list the carbon dioxide emissions value of foods. They've also drafted new dietary recommendations that take into account the environmental impact of diet.

Buying animal products from small mom-and-pop farms may be preferable to buying from large companies that engage in animal agriculture on a large scale. Small, local farmers often are more sensitive to environmental hazards associated with raising animals for food. However, in general, becoming less dependent on dairy and other animal products is best for everyone.

Taking a Closer Look at Ethical Considerations

Albert Schweitzer, the famous theologian, musician, physician, philosopher, and recipient of the Nobel Peace Prize, was once quoted as saying, "Until he extends his circle of compassion to all living things, man will not himself find peace." That remark pretty much sums up the rationale for some people who opt to live dairy-free (and meat-free). Basically, they avoid dairy out of a strong sense of ethics and compassion for animals.

Figuring out whether dairy-free also means meat-free

The ethical, environmental, and health reasons that some people go dairy-free apply just as well to the practice of eating meat. In fact, most people who go dairy-free for these reasons are already living meat-free. Here are the many effects of eating a meat-filled diet:

✔ **Ethical:** Animals raised for meat are, like dairy cows, confined to factory farms. They suffer, and their lives end violently in slaughterhouses, where conditions for the humans who work there are abysmal. To avoid causing pain and suffering to animals, many people advocate a vegetarian diet. Some famous veg-heads include Pythagoras, Socrates, Leonardo da Vinci, and Benjamin Franklin.

Many books have been written about the ethical issues surrounding the idea of eating animals and other animal products. Two examples include *Animal Factories,* which was revised and updated by Jim Mason and Peter Singer (Three Rivers Press), and *Farm Sanctuary: Changing Hearts and Minds About Animals and Food* by Gene Baur (Touchstone).

✔ **Environmental:** As I explain further in the section "Contemplating climate change," the meat and dairy industries collectively contribute substantially to problems with global warming. The meat industry also is a major polluter, affecting supplies of clean water, soil, and air.

✔ **Health related:** Many of the health reasons for going dairy-free apply equally to a meat-free diet. Like dairy products, meats are high in artery-clogging saturated fat, so meat-eaters have higher risks of coronary artery disease than people who don't eat meat. In fact, a large body of scientific research now supports the idea that vegetarian diets in general support good health. Vegetarians live longer than nonvegetarians, and they have lower risks for numerous chronic diseases and conditions, including high blood pressure and cholesterol, cancer, and diabetes. Vegetarians also often are slimmer.

You can find the American Dietetic Association's position paper on vegetarian diets at `www.eatright.org/WorkArea//DownloadAsset.aspx?id=8417`. And, of course, another good source of information is my book *Living Vegetarian For Dummies* (Wiley).

Does dairy-free also mean meat-free for you? It's possible. Decisions about diet are very personal. Give it some thought, and do what feels right for you.

Many people who go dairy-free do it as part of an ethical stance. They believe it's immoral to exploit animals for food that they don't need. They don't want to support the treatment that the animals receive in factory farms — or any farms, for that matter. They also don't want to drink milk and eat other dairy products because by doing so, they indirectly support the meat industry, including the inhumane treatment of male calves in the veal trade.

If you've ever shared your life with a dog or cat — or even a rat — you know that animals have feelings. They express excitement, happiness, fear, and anger. There's no mistaking the meaning of a wagging tail and nudge of a nose, or a yelp, meow, or squeak of excitement when a treat is offered or a dinner bowl is set out. Even if you don't share your home with a cow, it isn't difficult to imagine that like other mammals you know and love, cows have feelings, too. They may not look like your dogs, cats, or rats, but they feel pleasure and pain just the same.

Given the fact that animals have feelings, many people can't help but be upset with how unpleasant it is for dairy cows to live their lives confined to factory farms. They remain there until they're no longer of use. At that point, they're sent to the slaughterhouse where their lives end violently. Even animals raised on small, mom-and-pop farms where they have access to more space may have their lives ended violently.

For more information about the ethics concerning animal rights, go online to the People for the Ethical Treatment of Animals (PETA) Web site at www. peta.org.

Eyeing Economic and Political Forces that Keep Dairy in the American Diet

The U.S. Department of Agriculture (USDA) is charged with protecting and promoting American agriculture, which includes the meat and dairy industries. At the same time, the USDA also has the primary responsibility for revising and issuing the Dietary Guidelines for Americans (DGA) every five years. The DGA are the cornerstone of all federal nutrition programs, including the National School Lunch Program. The DGA are supposed to describe an optimal diet for keeping Americans healthy.

The problem is that the goal of protecting the meat and dairy industries is increasingly at odds with what science considers to be an optimal diet for humans. Most scientific evidence considers an optimal diet to be one that's low in animal products and high in plant matter. And, of course, that's a message the meat and dairy industries resist.

This conflict of interest has for many years made it difficult, if not impossible, for the USDA to reconcile the interests of the public's health with the interests of American *agribusiness* — the large, corporate factory farms. This built-in conflict has complicated the production of dietary recommendations and resulted in guidelines that were weak and unclear.

Fortunately, the most recent set of DGA is much improved over past years. In addition to acknowledging that some people may prefer to eat a vegetarian diet, mention also is made of alternatives to cow's milk for those who prefer to live dairy-free.

Still, the dairy industry influence remains evident in American food policy today and is responsible for keeping dairy products in the diets of many people. Fluid cow's milk, for example, is required to be served with every federally reimbursable meal in the National School Lunch Program. A doctor's note with a medical excuse is required for children to receive a nondairy alternative to cow's milk at lunchtime. And federal subsidies, price supports, and other economic incentives keep dairy products profitable to produce and sell.

 An excellent resource that goes into much more detail about the economic and political forces at work to keep dairy in your diet is the book, *Food Politics: How the Food Industry Influences Nutrition and Health* by Marion Nestle (University of California Press).

Going Dairy-Free with Some Restrictions

For some people, going dairy-free isn't as easy as it is for others because of their health. They may have allergies or other intolerances to foods commonly used to replace dairy products. In this section, I mention two examples.

When soy isn't an option

Soymilk is one product that's especially tasty, nutritious, and versatile to use in place of milk. And other soy products, including tofu, soy-based cheeses, soy coffee creamer, and soy ice cream are all great nondairy substitutes for dairy products, too. Unfortunately, soy isn't the best choice for everyone. Some people are allergic to soy. People with soy allergies may develop symptoms such as abdominal cramps, nausea, or diarrhea if they eat foods containing soy. The level of intolerance varies from person to person. A few tablespoons of soymilk or soy creamer in a cup of coffee may not bother one person, but the same amount may cause severe symptoms for the next person.

 Individuals with soy allergies should follow the advice of their healthcare providers or figure out through trial and error how much soy they can successfully include in their diets without causing discomfort. If you're allergic to soy, you may need to use other nondairy products that don't contain soy.

When almonds aren't an option

Like people with soy allergies, some people are allergic to tree nuts, including almonds. As a result, these individuals have to avoid almond milk, a product that's appearing more frequently in supermarkets as an alternative to cow's milk. They also have to avoid other nondairy products made from almonds, such as nondairy cheese and ice cream.

Fortunately, people with tree nut allergies can use many other nondairy products. Rice milk, for example, is hypoallergenic and can be used in place of almond milk.

 If you need help navigating your choices when you have food allergies, you may want to get individualized counseling from a registered dietitian or your healthcare provider.

Chapter 3

Dairy-Free by Degree: Taking a Look at Lactose Intolerance

*F*ood shouldn't make you hurt, right? For many people, though, a glass of milk with their cookies, a slice of pizza, or an ice cream cone are all it may take to send them to the bathroom with diarrhea or to bed with abdominal cramps. These uncomfortable symptoms often are due to lactose intolerance, a condition that stops people from being able to digest dairy products. Because of its symptoms, this condition is the most common reason people have for avoiding dairy products.

In this chapter, I describe the science behind lactose intolerance. I also explain what the symptoms are, who usually suffers from them, and why. I also help you determine how strict you need to be about avoiding dairy products and how to size up what it means for your lifestyle.

Getting the Lowdown on Lactose Intolerance

You may be surprised to discover that lactose intolerance is natural. In fact, most adult humans around the world are lactose intolerant to some extent. *Lactose intolerance* basically is an inability to digest the milk sugar *lactose*. The condition is caused when individuals don't produce enough *lactase*, the enzyme needed to digest lactose.

In the following sections, I describe how your body changes over time in its ability to digest milk, what happens when you no longer need milk, and how your body responds to dairy when you're intolerant. This section uncovers why some people can eat all the dairy products they want and why others have to watch every mouthful.

Knowing why lactose intolerance occurs

People tend to think of lactose intolerance as being something abnormal — a condition that needs special attention, like an illness or a disease. However, lactose intolerance is actually a natural state of being for most of the world's adults. Understanding what lactose intolerance is and why it happens, though, may change your perspective and make you better able to manage your diet and your symptoms. The following sections look at the evolution of lactose intolerance and its causes.

Examining milk: Nature's first food

For every mammal on Earth — including humans — milk is the first food they eat. A mammal's milk is tailor-made to be exactly what a baby mammal of that species needs. Squirrels, for example, produce milk that contains precisely what a baby squirrel needs to grow and develop normally. Dogs produce milk that's customized for their puppies. And cows feed their calves milk that's formulated to help a tiny calf grow into a hulking herbivore in little more than a few months.

Humans produce milk for their babies, too, and it's the optimal food for normal human growth and development. It's better than baby formula, and it's better for human babies than milk from a squirrel or a dog. No other mammal drinks the milk of another mammal species. So the question is why do humans drink milk from a cow? (The sidebar "Culture and the role of dairy in the diet" can shed some light on the answer.)

Because milk is for babies, mammal mothers only make it until their infants are nourished and have developed well enough to tolerate solid foods. Until then, a mother's milk provides her offspring with special substances that boost immunity and provide the calories, protein, carbohydrates, fat, vitamins, and minerals they need to grow.

One ingredient in a mother's breast milk is lactose, a form of sugar. A baby's body produces an enzyme — *lactase* — that's specially designed to help digest the lactose in milk. With the help of lactase, the body breaks down lactose into small forms of sugar — glucose and galactose — that are readily absorbed into the bloodstream and used to produce energy. Over time, though, babies grow and develop to the point where they can eat solid foods.

Gradually, they're weaned from breast milk. At that point, if they're squirrels, they start eating acorns. And dogs, like humans, begin eating a wide variety of foods. Cows start eating grass. When babies of all species no longer need their mothers' milk to survive, they stop producing lactase — at least most of them do.

Lactase deficiency — insufficient amounts of the enzyme lactase — also can be caused another way: It can result from damage to the small intestine, where lactase is produced, from such conditions as severe diarrhea, chemotherapy, radiation, Crohn's disease, and celiac disease (also known as *gluten-induced enteropathy*).

Lacking lactase results in lactose intolerance

By the time humans and other mammals reach adulthood, they generally don't produce lactase. So, if they drink milk or eat foods made from milk, they can't digest the lactose in the milk.

The waning of lactase production that begins in late childhood and extends into adolescence and adulthood is sometimes referred to as *lactase nonpersistence*.

This natural lack of lactase in turn causes *lactose malabsorption*. When lactose malabsorption results in symptoms, the condition is considered lactose intolerance. The symptoms of lactose intolerance can all be attributed to the undigested lactose moving through the gastrointestinal system. (Check out the next section for the symptoms caused by lactose intolerance.)

Identifying the symptoms

If you're lactose intolerant, your body can't digest the milk sugar lactose, leading to any of a number of unpleasant symptoms. When undigested milk sugars enter the colon, bacteria cause them to ferment and result in symptoms.

The symptoms of lactose intolerance are similar to the symptoms you may experience from time to time when you're sick, have a mild case of food poisoning, or ate something that didn't agree with you that day. Symptoms include the following:

- Abdominal cramps
- Bloating
- Diarrhea
- Gas
- Nausea

Culture and the role of dairy in the diet

After the Native Americans settled North America, Europeans did the same and brought with them their tradition — and tolerance — for eating dairy products. For the next couple hundred years, the customs and systems that developed favored this European-centric dietary preference. A powerful dairy industry evolved along with national agricultural policies. With these dairy-centered evolutions came such long-standing traditions as ice cream socials, the basic four food groups (with milk being one of the four pillars), mandatory cow's milk in school lunches, and milk mustache ads in magazines. Today, the dairy industry and related businesses, in collaboration with local, state or provincial, and federal governments continue to support the consumption of cow's milk for complex political and economic reasons.

You've probably experienced these problems at least occasionally. People who suffer from lactose intolerance, though, experience one or more of these symptoms often, especially after they've eaten a big dose of dairy. Some people suffer symptoms of lactose intolerance for years before making the connection between what they eat and how they feel.

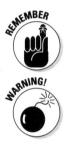

Lactose intolerance affects individuals differently. Even within families, one person's level of tolerance for lactose may be different than another's.

Don't assume you have lactose intolerance just because you have gas, bloating, nausea, abdominal cramps, or diarrhea. Other conditions, including irritable bowel syndrome, inflammatory bowel disease, and others, can cause similar symptoms. Your healthcare provider can help you make an accurate diagnosis. Also, don't confuse lactose intolerance with milk allergy. They're two different conditions. In milk allergy, the body has an immune response to proteins in cow's milk. This situation is more common in infants less than 1 year old, while lactose intolerance is more common in adolescents and adults.

Determining Your Degree of Intolerance

Every human has a unique genetic makeup, and many people have family trees with branches from various parts of the world. So it makes sense that some people may be more or less able to tolerate dairy in their diets. In fact, some individuals diagnosed with lactose malabsorption, low lactase levels, or who fit the genetic profile for having low lactase levels don't show symptoms of lactose intolerance — even when they're challenged with a big dose of dairy.

Figuring out the extent to which you tolerate dairy isn't clear-cut and easy. The good news is that I'm here to help. In the following sections, I show you how your family tree can affect your tolerance and also explain how you can hone in on where you stand on the intolerance scale.

Understanding the variations: Who is lactose intolerant and who isn't

Lactose malabsorption or intolerance doesn't affect everyone. In fact, up to about 25 percent of the world's adult humans can digest milk without problems. However, the breakdown on who's affected has many shades of gray. Think of lactose malabsorption and lactose intolerance as being on a continuum. (See Figure 3-1.)

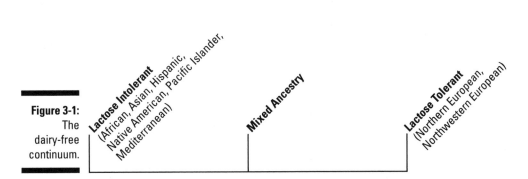

Figure 3-1:
The dairy-free continuum.

Lactose Intolerant
(African, Asian, Hispanic, Native American, Pacific Islander, Mediterranean)

Mixed Ancestry

Lactose Tolerant
(Northern European, Northwestern European)

On this spectrum are the following three main groups:

- **People who tolerate lactose in the diet very well:** These lactose lovers all have something in common: They have ancestors from northern or northwestern Europe — Ireland, Scotland, England, Wales, the Scandinavian countries, and others. They have the ability to produce the lactase needed to digest milk sugars and can eat dairy products freely.

  Scientists believe generations ago, people from these parts of the world developed a genetic mutation that allowed them to continue making lactase into adulthood. Long ago, many of these population groups were herders. The genetic mutation, or trait, they developed made it possible for them to drink the milk of the animals they raised. Over the generations, these Europeans passed this trait on to their descendents — mostly Caucasians — who today can eat a cheese sandwich or drink a milkshake without doubling over in pain.

- **People with little or no ability to produce lactase and digest dairy:** This group contains the 75 percent of folks who have little or none of the preceding European decent. Most Africans, Asians, Hispanics, Native Americans, Alaska Natives, Pacific Islanders, and people of Mediterranean descent fall into this category. For these individuals, even small amounts of milk or milk products may cause a range of unpleasant symptoms.

> ✔ **People who fall somewhere in-between:** These folks' dairy tolerances depend on their own unique genetic makeup. In some cases, people of mixed ancestry may be able to eat cheese on pizza or a cup of yogurt now and then. Adding a glass of milk or dish of ice cream at the same meal, though, may be too much and cause symptoms to develop. How much is too much simply depends on the individual.

A 2010 report on lactose intolerance and health by the National Institutes of Health concluded that it's impossible to accurately estimate the number of people in the United States who are affected by lactose malabsorption or lactose intolerance. In part, that's because studies have been inconsistent in the way they define the condition. The bottom line is that the majority of the world's adults are affected — whether they have symptoms or not — because many humans aren't designed to digest milk after infancy.

The number of lactose intolerant people in the United States is likely to grow in the coming years. Census data shows that the nonwhite minority in the United States is going to be a majority by the year 2050. People in this minority are the most likely to be lactose intolerant.

Testing for lactose intolerance

The symptoms of lactose intolerance are common for many other conditions, which is why it can't be diagnosed based on the symptoms alone (see the earlier section "Identifying the symptoms" for more information). So, the easiest way to test for lactose intolerance is a simple *elimination diet,* where you eliminate dairy foods. If you suspect that you're lactose intolerant, your doctor would likely suggest the same thing after asking you questions about your medical history and doing a physical exam.

Uncovering additional information

If you're curious and want to read more in-depth reports and findings about lactose intolerance, you can obtain additional information online from the following reliable sources:

✔ The National Institutes of Health Consensus Development Conference Statement on lactose intolerance and health is available at `consensus.nih.gov`.

✔ The National Digestive Diseases Information Clearinghouse (NDDIC) Web

site at `digestive.niddk.nih.gov/ddiseases/pubs/lactose intolerance` provides detailed information on symptoms, causes, and risks.

✔ The Mayo Clinic Web page on lactose intolerance at `www.mayoclinic.com/health/lactose-intolerance/DS00530` also is helpful for symptom, diagnosis, and risk-factor information.

The elimination diet is easy to try. To see whether you're lactose intolerant, just cut out all milk and dairy products, including foods made with milk or other dairy products, for a short period of time — a few days to a week. If your symptoms go away, you may have your answer. You may determine that certain foods bother you more than others. Check out the "Experimenting with your dairy limits" section for suggestions on how to find that middle ground.

Your doctor also may decide to conduct other tests to zero in on a diagnosis of lactose intolerance. These tests include the following:

- ✔ **A hydrogen breath test:** After drinking a high-lactose beverage, your breath is analyzed over a period of time to check the levels of hydrogen. People who produce lactase have less hydrogen in their breath. People who don't produce lactase and are lactose intolerant are more likely to have high levels of hydrogen in their breath. The hydrogen is caused when bacteria ferment the undigested lactose in the colon.

- ✔ **A stool acidity test:** If you don't produce lactase and can't digest lactose, acids and sugar can be detected in a stool sample. This test often is used for infants and young children experiencing digestive problems to help healthcare providers rule out various causes. *Remember:* Lactose intolerance is uncommon in infants and young children, but babies born prematurely may be affected.

- ✔ **Intestinal biopsy:** In this test, the doctor examines a small piece of your intestinal tissue and measures the level of lactase activity.

- ✔ **Genetic testing:** Scientists can use genetic testing to determine whether you have the genes associated with production of lactase in adulthood or the genes associated with lactase nonpersistence.

Experimenting with your dairy limits

You may discover that you can handle smaller amounts of dairy in your diet rather than cutting it completely. The most practical way to figure out how much dairy you can — or can't — tolerate is to experiment with your diet. You have various ways to experiment. For example, you can do the following:

- ✔ **Vary the amount of dairy you take in.** A full cup of milk may be too much for you to tolerate, but a few tablespoons of it in your coffee may be okay. By experimenting with different amounts of milk and milk products in your diet, you can zero in on your individual tolerance level.

- ✔ **Vary the type of dairy products you choose.** Some people find they can tolerate certain forms of milk or milk products better than others. For example, some people can digest yogurt or cheddar cheese, but they may develop symptoms when they drink milk or eat ice cream.

Yogurt with active cultures and hard cheeses, such as cheddar, Swiss and Parmesan, tend to be better tolerated than other forms of milk and soft cheeses, such as mozzarella and ricotta cheese. Active cultures in yogurt help to break down some of the lactose in milk, and hard cheeses — especially those that are aged for more than two years — contain much less lactose than many other types of cheese.

✔ **Gradually introduce dairy into your diet.** Completely remove milk and milk products from your diet, and then slowly add them back over a period of days or weeks. Introduce one product at a time so that you can more easily pinpoint the offender if symptoms arise.

Begin with small quantities at first, and then build up to more. Pay attention to signs that your symptoms are returning. When they do, you may have found your limit.

✔ **Spread out the dairy products that you consume.** Some people find they can tolerate more dairy products if they spread them out over the day, rather than eating a big dose at a single sitting. For example, they may be able to add milk to their coffee in the morning and eat a small amount of cheese on a baked potato at dinner. But if they put milk in their coffee and also eat a bowl of cereal with milk at the same meal, it may be enough to induce symptoms.

✔ **Dilute the dairy products with other foods.** Some people find that eating a small amount of a dairy product with other foods in a meal is better tolerated than eating the dairy product by itself. For example, rather than eating a chunk of cheese or drinking a glass of milk, they may tolerate the dairy product better by eating it in combination with a few crackers or a piece of toast.

What works for one person may not work for you. Testing various approaches can help you discover your tolerance limits for dairy as well as strategies for increasing those limits.

Putting the Dairy-Free Issue in Perspective

Limiting your intake of dairy products — or even avoiding them completely — can seem like a daunting task when you first consider it. Milk and foods made from milk are a deeply rooted tradition in North America and throughout most of Europe. Not only do these foods turn up in homes, stores, and restaurants everywhere, but they often play an important part in our social lives, too. For example, what's birthday cake without a scoop of ice cream? What about Grandma's brownie without a glass of milk?

Getting along without drinking or eating dairy products may take some adjustment. In this section, I suggest a few ideas to help you get your head around the change.

Considering dairy alternatives

As ubiquitous as dairy foods are today, you can find just as many dairy-free foods worthy of your attention and enjoyment. It's all a matter of how you look at things. You don't have to limit yourself. Rather you can look for other alternatives that are just as satisfying. For example, instead of an ice cream cone, have a frozen fruit bar, Italian ice, or a dish of sorbet. Or leave the cheese sauce off your nachos and enjoy some fresh salsa and guacamole to the fullest.

When looking to try alternatives, keep the following in mind:

✔ **Be aware of the changes you need to make.** Educating yourself — as you're doing by reading this book — is a good way to start. Keeping a food diary for a while also can be illuminating by helping you become more familiar with how you depend on dairy products. I discuss food diaries in more detail in Chapter 5.

✔ **Know how to make those changes.** As you consider your options, view the transition as a matter of reprogramming old habits. And know that you can make use of the tips and approaches I cover in this book. Get started with the advice in Chapter 5 for making the transition to a dairy-free diet. From there, Parts II and III give you the practical guidance you need to build dairy-free meals you can live with and love.

✔ **Get support to sidestep dairy products for the long run.** Many sources of support are available, including online groups, a registered dietitian who can give you individualized counseling, and friends who may be working on similar dietary changes. Part IV of this book focuses on the lifestyle workarounds that you need to consider, including navigating social situations, eating out, and managing a dairy-free diet in the context of your family life.

Over time, you can go dairy-free with ease. Some people find it helpful to document lifestyle changes in a journal, making daily entries that chronicle their challenges and discoveries along the way. If journaling appeals to you, you also may enjoy starting a blog on the Internet. Blogs are interactive, and other people can join in on the discussion by posting their own comments and questions. Two popular blog platforms are Blogger and Typepad. You can visit my blog at www.onthetable.net and join in the discussion!

Assessing the risks and rewards

Lifestyle change isn't easy, especially when it entails changing long-held habits or traditions. The risks you take in beginning to eliminate dairy products from your diet are similar to those you would encounter if you were trying to make other diet changes, including losing weight or going vegetarian.

Changing your diet takes time and planning. At times you'll make progress, and every once in a while, you may take a step backward, too. And sometimes you may feel discouraged or down, especially when you're busy or under pressure and the effort the new lifestyle requires feels like a burden.

Expect to experience a few times, too, when you feel a sense of social isolation due to your diet. You'll encounter times when the group wants to order pizza and yours needs to be cheese-free, or when your host serves a cheesecake and you have to settle for a cup of coffee — black.

Over time, the downsides to a dairy-free lifestyle will diminish as you gain skills and confidence about how to manage. When you get there, you'll know it. Handling your diet will become automatic and natural to you.

Of course, the benefits will be for your health. You'll feel better, and you'll have the added satisfaction of knowing you're also reducing your intake of saturated fat and protecting your heart. And the cherry on top is that you'll be making a contribution to preserving the environment and extending compassion to the cows, too.

It may also help to remind yourself from time to time that you're a human being, not a cow. In fact, you're an adult human, not a calf. Choosing to go dairy-free is compatible with your biology. If you were meant to drink cow's milk, you would have the capacity to digest it. In other words, you would be a cow. (To understand the biology behind digesting milk, check out the earlier section "Knowing why lactose intolerance occurs.")

Chapter 4

Getting Calcium, Vitamin D, and Other Essential Nutrients

....

....

*N*o one food has all the nutrients you need. That is, unless you're a baby. For infants, milk has everything a body needs to grow and develop into toddlerhood. By the second or third year of life, your body makes the transition away from breast milk to solid foods. These foods provide the dietary fiber and other nutrients not found in milk that are needed to support continued good health.

At that point, there's nothing in human breast milk that you need and can't get from other foods. If humans don't need human milk in childhood and later, they definitely don't need milk from a cow. So why would anybody advise you to drink it? The answer is complicated, but I try to lay out the nutritional rationale for drinking cow's milk — or not — in this chapter.

Furthermore, I explain the issues surrounding your need for calcium, vitamin D, and other essential nutrients that dairy products can provide. I also examine the arguments for and against taking supplements of these nutrients if you don't include cow's milk in your diet.

Understanding Why People Consume Dairy Products

Drinking cow's milk is like taking a liquid nutritional supplement. It's a concentrated source of calcium and a rich source of protein, riboflavin, potassium, vitamin B12, and other vitamins and minerals. It's the perfect food for transforming a 75-pound calf into a half-ton cow in a matter of months. Perhaps as a result, although cow's milk is meant for cows, humans have claimed it as a dietary pillar for generations.

Despite all the good nutrients it provides, milk also includes some things humans need to limit in their diets, such as sodium and saturated fat. Milk also is low or devoid in other necessary substances, such as dietary fiber, iron, and some of the beneficial *phytochemicals* (substances found in foods of plant origin, such as broccoli and beans).

For those who can digest cow's milk, a little bit of nonfat or low-fat milk in the diet is probably fine and provides a dose of nutrition. Too much, though, puts you at risk for displacing calories from foods that can provide other much-needed nutrients not found in cow's milk. Getting the balance right can be a challenge when you're raised in a cow's milk–happy culture.

Milk: A constant in meal planning advice over the years

Government guidelines for healthful eating have for many years perpetuated the idea that milk is a part of a balanced diet. You may remember the Basic Four Food Groups, which started as an industry marketing tool and was later adopted as a government meal-planning guide. Everyone was advised to eat foods from these four groups every day in order to achieve a so-called balanced diet. The Basic Four Food Groups have since been discarded and replaced by the MyPyramid planning tool.

A rainbow of fruits and vegetables made up one of the four original basic groups. A collection of breads and cereal grains made up another. Meats and other protein-rich foods were grouped together. And then there was milk. A single substance — cow's milk — was considered one of the four cornerstones of a healthful human diet. Of course, dairy products in this group included milk plus sugar and fat (ice cream and yogurt), milk plus salt and fat (cheese), milk fat (sour cream and whipped cream), and so on.

Cow's milk is still identified as a recommended food group in the U.S. Department of Agriculture MyPyramid food guide. However, the guide now advises choosing only nonfat and low-fat varieties of milk, yogurt, and cheese. After all, cow's milk is a food with nutritional pros and cons when consumed by humans.

The Big Kahuna: Calcium

Calcium is the one nutrient most associated with milk. When you hear recommendations to drink cow's milk, it's primarily because, where calcium is concerned, it's the mother lode.

Why all the fuss about calcium? Health professionals care about how much calcium you consume because it's so vital to your health. If you don't get enough calcium in your diet — or your body can't hang on to the calcium you already have — you may develop osteoporosis. *Osteoporosis* is a condition in which your bones become porous and brittle, allowing them to break easily. Some people with osteoporosis break bones simply by sneezing too hard or falling down. For older adults, these breaks can have life-threatening consequences.

So, naturally, doctors and nutritionists have long had people flocking to cow's milk to keep up their calcium levels. The calcium in cow's milk — and its relationship with bone health — is why milk has been given its status as a singular food group in dietary guidance tools. But bone health depends on far more than the amount of calcium in your diet.

In this section, I dig a little deeper into these issues to help you better understand your calcium needs — what the science says about your needs and why, where (besides cow's milk) you can get calcium in your diet, how to ensure you get enough, and how to hang on to what you've got.

Determining how much calcium you need

Building strong bones isn't as simple as eating lots of calcium. The science actually is much more complicated than that. A constellation of factors affects the amount of calcium you need from your diet as well as the amount that finally reaches — and stays in — your bones. Scientists do the best they can to estimate the effects of these factors when they issue dietary recommendations for the public.

Of course, those recommendations are for large populations of people. Because each person eats somewhat differently and has different lifestyle habits and genetic profiles, a person's individual calcium needs may be somewhat different than the recommendations made for the masses. When making general recommendations, though, scientists start by making a rough guess as to how much calcium humans need. Here's the process scientists take to estimate recommendations:

1. **They figure that each person loses a certain amount of calcium every day.**

   You lose calcium through your urine, feces, and even your sweat.

2. **They subtract that amount from the average amount of calcium you take in and absorb from your food each day.**

   They know the average amount of calcium people consume every day from national dietary surveys.

3. **With that information, scientists calculate the amount of calcium most people need each day from their diets to break even, considering the daily gains and losses.**

4. **They pad that final figure a little bit, just for good measure.**

Recommended levels of calcium intake for Americans vary by age and sex. Scientists (those who make recommendations) generally assume the worst, though, and try to compensate for the average American's poor eating habits.

Nutritionists don't really expect anyone to count the number of milligrams of calcium they eat every day. Instead, they suggest that you aim for some general meal planning guidelines. (I include meal-planning advice in Chapter 7.)

It bears repeating, though, that your individual needs vary, depending on a host of lifestyle and other factors. In this section, I describe them in more detail.

Sodium sense

Too much sodium can rob your body of its calcium stores. Unfortunately, most people get far more sodium in their diets than what's good for them.

Where do people get all this sodium? Just look around. Sodium is a major component of table salt, so any time you shake salt on your food, you're adding sodium. Of course, foods with lots of added salt — soup, pickles, popcorn at the theater, salty chips, and snack foods, for example — also are high in sodium. Processed foods are high in sodium as well. Examples include packaged rice mixes, pudding mixes, frozen entrees, processed meats and cheeses, condiments such as ketchup and soy sauce, and many fast foods.

Although the human body does need some sodium, the amount needed is small. And you can get all you need naturally from foods that have no added sodium or salt. No one has to *try* to get sodium — it's already there in the fresh carrots, celery, tomatoes, spinach, and other foods that grow in your garden.

The power of protein

Recent research on the relationships between protein and calcium intakes has shed new light on an old issue in nutrition. For many years, nutritionists warned that eating too much protein may increase the loss of calcium from bones. A careful review of the research, though, doesn't bear this out as a concern. Higher protein intakes appear to have a slight positive effect on bone strength but have little effect on the risk of breaking a bone. Similar results are seen regardless of the source of protein. Higher intakes of total protein, animal protein, and vegetable protein all appear to have little effect on bone health. The bottom line: Aim to get adequate amounts of protein and calcium in your diet for optimal bone health.

To help conserve your body's calcium, read food labels and choose foods that are as low as possible in sodium. Keep your total sodium intake below 2,000 milligrams each day. A target of 1,500 milligrams is even better.

Phosphorus facts

You can get too much *phosphorus* in your diet. Phosphorus is a mineral that in excess can cause you to lose calcium. Meats, milk, soft drinks, and the caffeine in coffee and tea are rich in phosphorus. The effect of phosphorus on your body's calcium stores isn't as great as that of sodium, but it makes sense to be aware of the potential effects and to moderate your intake of high-phosphorus foods.

Living a dairy-free lifestyle can help preserve your body's phosphorus levels, which may help protect your calcium stores. By now, you can probably see why a bacon double cheeseburger, fries, and a cola should make your bones hurt!

Phytates and oxalates, oh my!

Even if you eliminate dairy from your diet and plan to get your calcium from other sources, you still have to be aware of other substances that can affect your calcium intake. *Phytates* and *oxalates*, for example, are in plant foods. They can bind with calcium and prevent your body from absorbing the calcium in the foods that contain them.

Whole grains, nuts, and beans contain phytates. Spinach, Swiss chard, and rhubarb are examples of foods high in oxalates. The phytates and oxalates in these foods prevent your body from absorbing the calcium they contain.

The good news: A lot of other plant foods contain plenty of calcium that's well absorbed. In fact, some research suggests that the calcium in many plant foods is absorbed by your body better than the calcium in cow's milk. Good examples of some of these calcium sources include broccoli, Chinese cabbage, and kale. So getting your calcium from these nondairy sources is a smart choice.

Putting your weight on it

Weight-bearing exercise — activities like walking, hiking, dancing, and lifting weights — helps you hang onto calcium. People who regularly engage in weight-bearing exercises like these have denser bones than people who don't. So for bone health, working these activities into your daily routine is a smart idea.

Sunlight matters

Have you ever heard the saying, "Vitamin D is the sunshine vitamin?" It's true. When your skin is exposed to sunlight, your body produces vitamin D, which is actually a hormone. Vitamin D has a key role in helping your body absorb calcium. I discuss vitamin D in more detail in the "Vitamin D: The Add-On" section later in this chapter. The important thing to know is that having enough vitamin D is important to bone health.

Adaptation

Your body can adapt when it needs to. In other words, depending on your dietary conditions, your body may be able to absorb more or less calcium from the foods you eat. For example, if your diet is short on calcium and you need it, your body may be able to absorb more. If you need less and you flood your body with calcium, you'll absorb less. Your body is a smart machine. But don't let that fact change your mind about whether you need to eat healthfully!

Identifying (dairy-free) food sources of calcium

Finding nondairy foods that contain plenty of calcium isn't difficult. In fact, many nondairy foods have calcium, so make sure you eat them often. Remember that horses, elephants, cows, and giraffes get all the calcium they need to build their massive skeletons by eating nothing more than plants (after the species-specific milk they drink in infancy, of course).

Table 4-1 lists the calcium content of some common nondairy sources of calcium. You don't need to count the milligrams of calcium in your diet.

However, you may find that a quick scan of this table helps you get a feel for how rich in calcium some foods are compared with others.

Table 4-1	Calcium Found in Nondairy Foods
Food	*Calcium Content (milligrams)*
1 medium artichoke, boiled	25
1 cup cooked lentils	38
1 tablespoon almond butter	43
1 flour or corn tortilla (6-inch)	45
2 slices whole-wheat bread	60
1 medium orange	61
1 cup cooked broccoli	62
1 cup canned garbanzo beans	77
1 tablespoon blackstrap molasses	82
1 cup canned kidney beans	87
1 cup cooked kale	94
1 ounce nondairy sour cream	100
1 cup canned pinto beans	103
1 cup cooked mustard greens	104
½ cup dried figs	121
1 cup canned navy beans	123
1 cup baked beans	126
2 tablespoons tahini	128
1 cup cooked bok choy	158
1 ounce soy mozzarella-style cheese	183
3 ounces salmon with bones	188
1 cup fortified almond milk	200
1 ounce fortified soy cheese	200
1 cup cooked turnip greens	209
1 cup cooked collard greens	266
1 6-ounce container soy yogurt (vanilla)	299
1 cup calcium-fortified orange juice	300
1 cup fortified rice milk	300
1 cup fortified soymilk	300
½ cup firm tofu (processed with calcium sulfate)	434

Even if you don't drink milk or eat other dairy products, it's not difficult to pack plenty of calcium into your meals. The following are healthful examples of calcium-rich meals, snacks, or dishes. Figure 4-1 also shows some examples:

- Whole-grain cereal with fortified soymilk and fresh berries
- Falafel (garbanzo bean balls) in pita pockets with plain soy yogurt sauce and a glass of fortified orange juice
- Bowl of navy bean soup with a fresh orange
- Black bean soup with a dollop of nondairy sour cream on top
- Stir-fried Chinese vegetables with pan-fried tofu over rice
- Fig cookies with a glass of fortified rice milk
- Black-eyed peas over rice with cooked collard greens
- Bowl of bean chili with steamed broccoli and nondairy cornbread
- Almond butter sandwich on whole-wheat toast

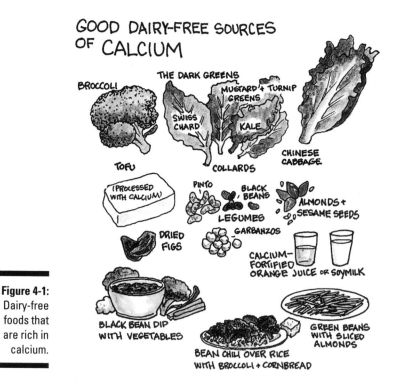

Figure 4-1:
Dairy-free foods that are rich in calcium.

Vitamin D: The Add-On

After calcium, vitamin D is the nutrient most associated with cow's milk. If you don't drink milk, where do you get your vitamin D? Good question. In this section, I explain the importance of vitamin D to health, how it got into your milk, and where to get it if you go dairy-free.

Getting the 4-1-1 on vitamin D and your body

Here's a news flash: Vitamin D isn't just a vitamin! It's also a hormone. A *hormone* is a chemical messenger produced by your body that sends messages that help to regulate the actions of cells or organs in the body.

So your body makes your own vitamin D and uses it to regulate other bodily functions. One of those functions is to regulate your body's calcium balance, which is necessary for proper mineralization of your bones. Your body is programmed to make and store vitamin D when your skin is exposed to sunlight.

Exposure to summer sunshine allows you to produce and store enough vitamin D to carry you through the winter months when there's less sunshine and you produce less vitamin D.

However, sometimes people find it difficult to get their daily dose of summer sunshine, which leads to a decreased production of vitamin D. I explain the reasons and risk factors and the symptoms of a vitamin D deficiency in the following sections.

Symptoms of a vitamin D deficiency

As noted earlier, not everybody gets the sunshine they need. In today's modern world, a lot of people — including me, sitting behind a computer writing this book — spend a great deal of time working indoors, where they have no exposure to summer sunshine. When you don't get enough vitamin D, you may notice symptoms, including bone pain and muscle weakness. Those symptoms usually are subtle, though, and you may not notice them until the vitamin deficiency becomes more severe.

Young children who don't get enough vitamin D can end up with *rickets,* a condition characterized by a softening and deformity of the bones.

Reasons you may not make enough vitamin D

People find that they can't make enough vitamin D for many reasons, including a limited exposure to sunlight. The reasons you may not get enough sunlight include the following:

- ✔ **You live in a smog-filled city.** If you live in a city that has a lot of air pollution, sunlight may be partially blocked.

- ✔ **You live in a Northern latitude.** If you live in the North, the sun's rays are less direct and summertime is shorter. You have less time to build up your vitamin D stores for the winter.

- ✔ **You live in a nursing home or you're housebound.** If you stay indoors — and this includes not only the elderly and infirm but also young, healthy people who simply work and play indoors most of the day — you limit your exposure to sunlight.

- ✔ **You cover up.** You hear a lot of health messages about the importance of using sunscreen to prevent skin cancer. But covering up with sunscreen and clothing has a downside — it may prevent you from getting enough sunlight to produce the amount of vitamin D you need to stay healthy.

You may be at increased risk of vitamin D insufficiency for other reasons, too. They include the following:

- ✔ **Having dark skin:** If you're Caucasian, you need about 5 to 30 minutes of direct summer sun on your hands and face at least twice a week between the hours of 10 a.m. and 3 p.m. when the sun's rays are most direct. People with dark skin may need even more (though precise guidelines aren't available). So they're at an even greater risk of not making enough vitamin D when they encounter the preceding conditions that limit their sunlight exposure. (Even so, African-Americans have lower rates of bone fracture from osteoporosis when compared with Caucasians.)

- ✔ **Growing older:** As you age, your body's ability to produce vitamin D diminishes. People over the age of 50 aren't as efficient at producing vitamin D in their skin, and the kidneys are less efficient at converting vitamin D to its hormone form.

- ✔ **Breastfeeding without a vitamin D supplement:** Babies who are breastfed and don't receive a vitamin D supplement may be at increased risk for a deficiency, especially if they have limited exposure to sunshine, wear sunscreen when they're outdoors, or are always covered up with clothing.

If you couple your body's natural decline in vitamin D production with any of the preceding risk factors and either of the following two factors, you may greatly increase your risk of vitamin D insufficiency:

- **Fat malabsorption:** Vitamin D is a *fat-soluble vitamin,* which means that it requires a certain amount of fat in your gastrointestinal system in order to be absorbed. If you have certain conditions, such as Crohn's disease, liver disease, or cystic fibrosis, difficulties absorbing dietary fat may limit your body's ability to absorb vitamin D, too.

- **Obesity or gastric bypass surgery:** If your Body Mass Index (BMI) is greater than or equal to 30, the extra fat layer under your skin may hinder release of vitamin D from your skin into the rest of your body. If you're obese and have gastric bypass surgery, the surgery bypasses the upper portion of the small intestine, which is where vitamin D is absorbed. This may lead to vitamin D insufficiency.

Body Mass Index (BMI) is a method of assessing your level of body fat based on your height and weight. The formula applies to both men and women. If you would like to calculate your BMI, try using the handy online BMI calculator at www.nhlbisupport.com/bmi.

As you can see, getting enough vitamin D can be a challenge for many people. In the next section, I tell you what the government did to help.

Seeing how vitamin D got into your milk

Because getting enough exposure to sunlight to produce the vitamin D you need can be difficult, the U.S. government put public health measures into place to add a layer of protection. Like putting fluoride in the water to prevent dental cavities, public health officials decided it would be a good idea to *fortify,* or add vitamin D to, foods that almost everyone consumed regularly.

In the United States, fluid cow's milk is routinely fortified with vitamin D. Orange juice, margarine, and breakfast cereals also may be fortified. Other dairy products, including ice cream, yogurt, cheeses, and sour cream, however, aren't typically fortified. In Canada, milk and margarine are required to be fortified with vitamin D.

Vitamin D fortification of foods is carefully regulated, because too much vitamin D can potentially be a problem. Because vitamin D is a fat-soluble vitamin and is stored in the body, excessively high intakes may be toxic.

The good news: You can go dairy-free and still get vitamin D with fortified nondairy products. With the rise in popularity of nondairy beverages such as soymilk and rice milk, brands that are fortified with calcium also are fortified with vitamin D to make them similar in nutrition to cow's milk.

Naming alternative sources of vitamin D

Finding alternative sources of vitamin D isn't easy. Very few foods are natural sources. Those that are include eggs and fatty fish, such as tuna, salmon, and sardines. So, other than making your own vitamin D from sunshine exposure or possibly getting some from the few food sources that naturally exist, your best bet for getting a dietary source of vitamin D is to eat fortified foods. Taking a vitamin D supplement also is an option, and I discuss that in more detail in the later section "Making Sense of Supplements."

Liver is a source of vitamin D, too, but it's not a good idea to eat it. An animal's liver is where environmental contaminants are deposited. You need vitamin D, but you sure don't need a big dose of contaminants along with it.

Obtaining what your body needs

Recommendations for vitamin D intake have gotten a lot of scrutiny by scientists lately. Current recommendations are for adults up to 50 years old to get 200 international units (IU) each day. People ages 51 to 70 should get double that amount, and people age 70 and older need 600 IU each day.

Recently, the American Academy of Pediatrics doubled the amount of vitamin D it recommends for children from 200 IU to 400 IU per day. The reason for the increase is growing scientific evidence that adequate vitamin D not only protects bones but may decrease the risk of other diseases, including cancer, multiple sclerosis, and diabetes.

If you know your exposure to sunlight is limited and you aren't confident that you're getting enough vitamin D from fortified foods, check in with your healthcare provider or a registered dietitian for individualized advice. Your physician may advise a blood test to determine whether your vitamin D level is adequate. You may need a supplement. I talk about supplements in more detail in the later section "Making Sense of Supplements."

Pinpointing Other Essential Nutrients in Milk

Like most foods, cow's milk is made up of a mix of nutrients. You need to get some of these nutrients from your diet whether you drink cow's milk and eat other dairy products or you decide to go dairy-free and get them from other sources. In this section, I run through a few of the other nutrients found in cow's milk that are of interest in human health.

Comprehending what your body needs

You need a wide range of vitamins, minerals, and other nutrients from foods to be healthy. Even though you don't need milk from a cow to be healthy, cow's milk does contain some nutrients (in addition to calcium and vitamin D) that support human health, including riboflavin, vitamin B12, and others.

If you don't want to or can't drink cow's milk or eat other dairy products, you're still okay nutrition wise. You can get the nutrients you need from plenty of other foods. I explain everything you need to know in the following sections.

Riboflavin

Riboflavin, which also is known as vitamin B2, is responsible for many functions in your body, chief among them helping enzymes initiate certain chemical reactions. Symptoms of a deficiency of riboflavin include a sore tongue, cracked and sore lips and corners of the mouth, and red, itchy eyes.

Dairy products are good sources of riboflavin, but many other sources are available, too. Meats (including organ meats) and eggs are a few examples, but you can opt for healthier choices as well.

Dairy-free sources of riboflavin that are healthiest for you overall include almonds, asparagus, bananas, beans, broccoli, figs, fortified soymilk and breakfast cereals, kale, lentils, mushrooms, peas, seeds, tahini, sweet potatoes, tempeh (a soy food), tofu, and wheat germ.

Vitamin B12

Like riboflavin, you need vitamin B12 for the proper functioning of enzymes that play critical roles in promoting normal metabolism. You need only a teeny-tiny amount of vitamin B12, but that teeny-tiny amount is vitally important. Deficiencies can cause a form of anemia and *neuropathy* (damage to the nerves in your hands, legs, feet, spinal cord, and brain).

Vitamin B12 is found only in animal products. If you don't drink milk or eat dairy products, you can get vitamin B12 from meats, seafood or fish, and poultry. If you don't eat any animal products at all, you can get vitamin B12 from fortified foods, such as vitamin B12–fortified soymilk, rice milk, and breakfast cereals. Or you can take a vitamin B12 supplement. (I discuss supplements in more detail later in this chapter.)

Assorted others

Cow's milk also contains phosphorus, potassium, selenium, and other vitamins and minerals. All these elements have roles in maintaining your health.

Knowing where to get what you need

Fortunately, you have many ways to get what you need from foods. A variety of diet approaches can work, with or without cow's milk and other dairy products.

The healthiest foods for humans include fruits, vegetables, whole-grain breads and cereals, beans and peas, and nuts and seeds. These foods contain the substantial amounts of dietary fiber, vitamins, minerals, protein, complex carbohydrates, and fats that you need to be healthy. Whether or not you eat dairy products, including a wide variety of these foundation foods in your diet — and getting enough calories to meet your energy needs — are two ways you can help ensure you'll get all the nutrition your body needs.

I provide two examples in Chapter 7 of meal planning guides you may find useful in pinning down exactly what you should eat to be healthy on a diet that omits cow's milk and other dairy products.

Making Sense of Supplements

Some people see vitamin and mineral *supplements* — concentrated doses of individual nutrients — as little daily servings of nutritional insurance. That may be an accurate perception for people who consistently eat diets that are heavy on the junk and light on the fruits, vegetables, whole grains, and legumes (which are important ingredients in a high-quality diet). For people who don't eat well, a multivitamin and mineral supplement may be useful in filling in the gaps.

Relying on supplements isn't ideal, though. After all, they aren't a sure thing (though they may be indicated in some circumstances). Plus, nutritional supplements can never really take the place of whole foods, which contain the full complement of nutrients you need for health. At best, they're a fallback position. At worst, they can hurt you. Still, whether or not you include dairy products in your diet, if you don't eat well consistently, you may need vitamin and mineral supplements. If you do take nutritional supplements, you should be sure to get good advice about what and how much to take.

In this section, I help you sort out the pros and cons of taking a vitamin or mineral supplement.

Taking a look at what the science says

Although nutritional supplements are used by many people (you probably have at least one bottle of vitamins or minerals in your medicine cabinet right now), you would be surprised to discover that their efficacy is far from certain. In fact, the evidence for the healthfulness of individual vitamins and minerals comes primarily from studies of those nutrients when they're packaged in whole foods and eaten as part of a typical diet — not when they're taken in supplement form.

Some scientists think that nutrients have a *synergistic* effect on each other. That is, they think certain nutrients need others to be present in the diet at the same time in order for you to get their full benefits. In general, claims about the health benefits of supplements have been greatly exaggerated by the multibillion dollar supplement industry.

The Institute of Medicine of the National Academies has reported, for example, that scientific evidence doesn't support health claims for some of the most popular supplements in recent years, including vitamins C and E, selenium, and beta carotene. And in a study published in 2009 in the *Archives of Internal Medicine*, 160,000 older women who took vitamin and mineral supplements had no significant differences in their risks of death, heart disease, and certain forms of cancer when compared with women who didn't take supplements.

In most cases, although their efficacy isn't certain, supplements won't hurt you. At other times, though, supplements can cause you harm. High doses of some nutrients, for example, can have unintended consequences. In an ordinary diet, nutrients usually balance each other out. But when you take concentrated doses of individual vitamins or minerals, one nutrient may interact with another. If you take too much zinc, for example, you may upset your body's balance of copper.

In the worst cases, vitamin and mineral supplements can increase your risk of health problems. For example, researchers found that people such as smokers, who are at high risk for lung cancer, may actually increase their risk of getting lung cancer when they take supplements of beta carotene, a form of vitamin A. (Beta-carotene from whole foods, though, appears to be safe.) Even vitamin E has been found in some studies to increase the risk of death when it's taken in high doses. The moral of the story is that you should talk with your healthcare provider before starting any new vitamin or mineral regimen.

Assessing your needs

Say you're living dairy-free and wondering whether you're getting the calcium, vitamin D, riboflavin, and other nutrients you need. Should you take a supplement?

You may not want to rely on nutritional supplements to get what you need (I explain why earlier in the chapter). Still, sometimes health professionals may think that taking one does make sense. It may not be optimal, but it may be the best option you have.

Here are a few of the situations in which taking a supplement may be better than not:

- ✔ **You're a strict vegetarian or vegan.** If you consistently eat a vegetarian diet that excludes meat, fish, and poultry — or a vegan diet that excludes meat, fish, poultry, eggs, milk, and other dairy products — you should consider a vitamin B12 supplement. After all, the only reliable sources of vitamin B12 that don't come from an animal are vitamin B12 supplements or foods fortified with vitamin B12, such as fortified soymilk or rice milk and fortified breakfast cereals.

  Vegans also may benefit from supplements of vitamin D, calcium, and possibly *docosahexaenoic acid* (DHA), an omega-3 fatty acid that's essential for human health.

  All vegheads can benefit from additional information in my book *Living Vegetarian For Dummies* (Wiley).

- ✔ **You're pregnant.** When you're eating for two, your healthcare provider may advise you to take a prenatal supplement as a form of health insurance, to fill in any gaps in your diet. I cover this topic in detail in Chapter 17.

- ✔ **You're breastfeeding a baby.** Breastfeeding puts extra demands on your body. Just like during pregnancy, your healthcare provider may recommend a supplement during this time to help ensure you're getting all the nutrients you need. I discuss this issue further in the section on vitamin D earlier in this chapter, and I also cover it in more detail in Chapter 17.

✔ **You're an older adult.** As you age, you need fewer calories than when you were younger. That leaves less room for sweets and other empty-calorie foods. Because eating well consistently is challenging, taking a supplement may be a way to hedge your nutritional bets. See the earlier section on vitamin D, or flip to Chapter 19 for more information.

Locating individualized advice

If you're living dairy-free and uncertain that you're meeting your nutritional needs, get some individualized advice before starting supplements. The most appropriate resource for nutrition counseling is a *registered dietitian* (RD). An RD is someone who has expertise in food and nutrition and has met specific educational and experience criteria set forth by the Commission on Dietetic Registration. Registered dietitians have passed a national registration exam and complete continuing education requirements.

You can ask your physician or other healthcare provider to refer you to a registered dietitian for a consultation. Dietitians often are associated with hospitals, but your physician may refer you to one who will see you on an outpatient basis. Some dietitians also are in private practice. You can find a registered dietitian on your own as well. Find one near you by contacting the American Dietetic Association's online referral service at www.eatright.org.

Chapter 5

Making the Transition to Dairy-Free: Getting Started

*F*or most people, drinking milk and eating dairy products have been ways of life since they were young. So making the switch to a diet without dairy may pose some challenges. After all, change is difficult. The good news is that despite the challenges, you can do it, and I explain how to get started transitioning to a dairy-free diet in this chapter.

First you have to be aware of the major dairy products you eat every day, and then you have to figure out how to avoid them. The next level of awareness includes understanding which foods contain less-obvious sources of dairy ingredients and starting to avoid those, too. Drafting a plan for a step-wise approach is a good idea when beginning to eliminate dairy products. This plan can help you track your progress and understand where to get help if you get stuck.

In addition, you also have to consider some other practical issues. For example, you need to be familiar with how to identify dairy ingredients on food labels and how to work with food company representatives to get answers to questions that may not be clear from those labels.

Finally, any major dietary change means knowing how to shop for alternatives, communicating your preferences to family and friends, and managing your food choices in social situations, including eating out. And you have to do all of this without losing your sense of humor — or your appetite! But don't worry, I guide the way in this chapter.

Spotting the Dairy in Your Diet

Going dairy-free means you have to omit milk, cheese, ice cream, sour cream, yogurt, and other dairy products from your diet. Easy enough, right? Not necessarily. Before you can omit the dairy and replace it with nondairy products, you first have to spot the dairy products.

After you detect the dairy, you have to determine how you want to replace the obvious sources. When you think about it, you probably put milk, cheese, and other dairy ingredients in a large number of the foods you eat every day. For example, there's the milk on your cereal, the shredded cheese on your nachos, and the melted mozzarella and ricotta layered in your lasagna.

Other sources of dairy are more difficult to see, however. Some are components of dairy products added as minor ingredients in many processed foods. Casein in margarine or soy cheese is one example. Skim milk solids added to a loaf of bread or ready-made piecrust is another.

In this section, I point out some of the most common sources of dairy you may be including in your diet right now as well as some sources that may not have occurred to you.

Identifying the usual suspects

You're probably familiar with the main dairy culprits. Just walk through any grocery store refrigerator dairy section, and you can see most of them. To get a clearer idea of what these products are, take a mental inventory of all the ways you use dairy products in your diet. Better yet, write them down on paper! A good way to start is to run through the list of most common dairy foods one at a time, thinking about all the dishes each ingredient is used to make.

For example, think about the many ways you use the following products:

- ✔ **Cheese:** You may use it to make grilled cheese sandwiches or cheeseburgers, to melt over your broccoli or nachos, to eat with crackers, and to sprinkle over your pasta or salads.

- ✔ **Cow's milk:** You may use it to make pancakes and cookies (and to dunk your cookies into!), cream soups, macaroni and cheese, homemade ice cream, yeast rolls, and pudding. You also may pour it over your cereal or in your coffee.

- ✔ **Ice cream:** You likely enjoy cake and ice cream, ice cream floats, ice cream cones and sundaes, milk shakes, and scoops straight from the carton.

- ✔ **Sour cream:** You probably top baked potatoes, pierogies (which themselves aren't always dairy-free), burritos, and nachos with this popular dairy product. You also may use it to make dips, cheesecake, or baked goods.

- ✔ **Yogurt:** It's a popular snack, and you may use it to bake, to top a burrito, or to make a granola parfait or smoothie.

I list other common dairy products in Chapter 6. After you take stock of what you're eating, you can begin to devise a plan for finding alternatives and working them into your routine.

Finding hidden sources of dairy

Depending on your level of sensitivity to the many components of dairy products, such as milk protein or milk sugar (lactose) — or how strict you want to be about omitting dairy from your diet — you may need to identify small amounts of these ingredients that sneak into your diet. For some people, even these tiny bits matter. In this case, it's especially important for you to do a good review of what you eat and to examine those foods for dairy-based ingredients.

Finding those dairy-based ingredients can be tricky. Byproducts of milk protein include

- ✔ **Casein (or caseinate):** Find it added to nondairy creamers, nutrition bars, salad dressings, whipped toppings, breath mints, and some soy cheeses.

- ✔ **Lactalbumin:** Find this protein added to baked goods, snack foods, textured vegetable protein products, and other processed foods.

- ✔ **Whey:** This liquid plasma portion of cow's milk is used in crackers, breads, processed cheeses, and other processed foods.

Other milk byproducts are made from the milk sugar lactose. They include saccharum lactin and D-lactose, which are used as a culture medium to sour milk. They're also used in processed foods, such as baby formula, desserts, and other sweets. In addition to foods, you also may find these ingredients in medicines, such as diuretics and laxatives.

A large number of processed foods contain dairy products or byproducts. The following list shows you some of the less-obvious foods that may contain dairy:

- Baby formula
- Baked goods
- Baking mixes
- Bircher muesli (Swiss granola cereal made with cream)
- Biscuits
- Breading on fried foods
- Breads
- Breakfast cereals
- Breath mints
- Candy
- Caramel
- Chocolate
- Chocolate drink mixes
- Coffee creamers (even some nondairy varieties)
- Cookies
- Crackers
- Cream liqueurs
- Ghee (clarified butter)
- Granola bars
- Gravy
- Instant potatoes
- Margarine
- Reduced-lactose milks, such as Lactaid
- Sherbet
- Soy cheese
- Whipped toppings

Make sure you read food ingredient labels carefully to spot some of these hidden sources of dairy. I include more label-reading advice in the "Reading ingredient labels" section later in this chapter.

Taking a Systematic Approach to Going Dairy-Free

Lifestyle changes can seem daunting to make. Like any large project you may take on, thinking about the task in its entirety can be overwhelming. That's why it helps to create a plan of attack and break down the task into more manageable chunks.

There's no right or wrong way to break down your plan to go dairy-free. It's all a matter of what feels right to you and how quickly you can adjust to the change. In this section, I help you come up with a plan that's right for you.

Outlining simple steps to de-dairy your diet

As you attempt to de-milk your diet, I suggest you work in small steps. Think about a series of logical steps you can take as you make the transition to a dairy-free lifestyle. As you master each step, you gain a sense of accomplishment that can help to keep you motivated as you continue.

Do anticipate a few bumps in the road as you make the transition, however. These challenges are a natural part of any big change. As you gain experience, you'll gain confidence. You'll also continue to discover and practice new meal-planning skills. A dairy-free lifestyle will become easier with time.

To create a plan with simple steps, write down what you want to do in a notebook, on a calendar, or on an erasable board. Tailor your plan to your own needs. For example, consider this sample list of steps that you may come up with:

> *Step 1:* Read this book cover to cover before doing anything else. Read some other resources, too, so I feel educated about the topic before going any further.

> *Step 2:* Cut out obvious sources of dairy and give myself a month to get used to that before refining my diet further.

> *Step 3:* Try my hand at new recipes and practice modifying some of my old favorites.

> *Step 4:* Begin eating out more often so I get used to handling social situations that involve meals away from home.

Just think about what the major steps will be for you and in what order you'd like to tackle them. Then sketch it out in a timeline. In Table 5-1, I outline one suggested approach for going dairy-free over a 12-week period of time. Follow this plan as is or modify it to suit your needs.

Table 5-1	Twelve Weeks to a Dairy-Free Eating Style
Time Frame	*What to Do*
Weeks 1 and 2	Read about dairy-free nutrition, meal planning, dealing with social situations, and other aspects of living dairy-free. Borrow books from the library, buy a few good resources at a bookstore, and check out online blogs and other materials on the Web. Soak up information and gain knowledge about this new lifestyle.
Week 3	Begin to reduce your intake of dairy products. Go dairy-free for two or three days this week, experiment with new products, and make a list of some of the dairy-free entrees and other foods you already enjoy.
Weeks 4 through 6	Cut back even more on your intake of milk and dairy products. Plan five dairy-free days each of these weeks. After Week 4, stop buying milk and other dairy products, and replace them with nondairy alternatives (if you haven't already). In order to gauge your progress later, keep a diary or log of everything you eat for several days.
Weeks 7 and 8	Get some support. Look for opportunities to socialize with people you know will make it easy on you. These are people who will be sympathetic and accommodating and won't give you grief for taking a step out of the mainstream. Continue reading and absorbing information and experimenting with new recipes. Go out to eat and order dairy-free meals at restaurants.
Weeks 9 through 12	Practice new skills and continue to educate yourself. Socialize and invite friends and family members to your home for dairy-free meals. Think about the past several weeks, and evaluate how you've handled various occasions. If you need more practice to master certain situations, such as eating away from home or finding quick and easy meal ideas, work on those. Keep a food diary for several days and compare it to your first one to see how far you've come.

Don't be discouraged if you have a lapse now and then in your new eating style. Slip-ups happen. They're especially likely when you have a break in your routine, such as when you're on vacation, when you're trying to survive the holidays, or when you get into a particularly hectic time at work or at home.

When you're under stress or you have an interruption in a new routine, it's natural to fall back into familiar lifestyle patterns. If this happens to you, don't dwell on your lapse. Just pick up where you left off and get back into your new eating style as soon as you can. Move on from there and don't look back.

Using a food diary

A *food diary* is a simple concept, but it's as helpful as can be. What does a food diary do? It helps you monitor what you've eaten and when. Basically it tells you a lot about where you are and where you need to go with your lifestyle change. At some point, it also will serve as an objective tool for gauging your progress, showing you just how far you've come over time. So, when you're transitioning to a dairy-free diet, consider keeping a food diary as you work on changing your eating style.

Creating a food diary is easy. Here's what to do:

✔ **Write down everything you eat or drink every day for a period of several days, a week, or however long you can stand it.** Use a notebook, index cards, a journal, or a word-processing document on your computer — whatever works for you and your lifestyle.

Maintaining your food diary on a notepad or small journal is convenient because you can tuck it into your purse or briefcase and have it handy whenever you need to make a quick note. However, online food diaries also are available. The advantage to these is that they can tally up your total daily calorie intake and analyze the nutritional value of your diet. One example I like is MyFoodDiary.com, which can be found online at www.myfooddiary.com. Or use your favorite Web browser to find another. Many are available, and they're easy to find with a simple Web search.

✔ **Keep your notes as detailed as possible.** If you have a bowl of cereal for breakfast, note whether you covered it with cow's milk or nondairy milk. If you ate a sandwich for lunch, note what the filling was and whether it contained cheese or any other dairy products.

Estimate portion sizes to the best of your ability, and jot those down as well. For example, note whether you had one cup of milk on your cereal, two slices of bread with your sandwich, a half cup of cooked vegetables with one teaspoon of margarine, and so on. This information may be useful at some point in helping you or a healthcare provider determine your level of sensitivity to milk protein or lactose.

✔ **Record what you eat as soon as you finish your meal or snack.** That way, you're less likely to forget to record — or to forget what you ate! Some people record at the end of each day, but don't fall into that habit. Your records will be more accurate if you record immediately after eating or drinking.

A typical food diary (for someone who's already dairy-free) may look like the one in Figure 5-1.

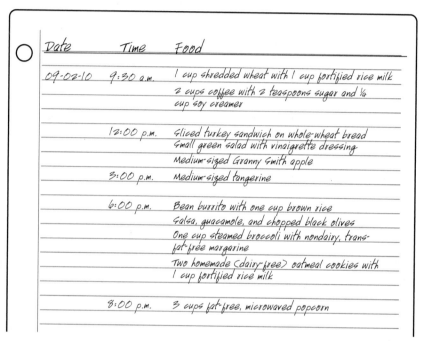

Date	Time	Food
09-02-10	9:30 a.m.	1 cup shredded wheat with 1 cup fortified rice milk
		2 cups coffee with 2 teaspoons sugar and ¼ cup soy creamer
	12:00 p.m.	Sliced turkey sandwich on whole-wheat bread
		Small green salad with vinaigrette dressing
		Medium-sized Granny Smith apple
	3:00 p.m.	Medium-sized tangerine
	6:00 p.m.	Bean burrito with one cup brown rice
		Salsa, guacamole, and chopped black olives
		One cup steamed broccoli with nondairy, trans-fat-free margarine
		Two homemade (dairy-free) oatmeal cookies with 1 cup fortified rice milk
	8:00 p.m.	3 cups fat-free, microwaved popcorn

Figure 5-1:
A food diary
for a single
day.

Monitoring your progress

Use your food diary to check your progress from time to time (see the preceding section to find out how to create a diary). After you've kept a food diary for an initial week or two, set it aside. Let several weeks go by, and then maintain a diary again for several days. Compare it to your first diary to see how far you've come. It can be motivating to see that you've consistently replaced cow's milk on your morning cereal with soymilk, that you're depending on fewer cheese-laden meals, and that when you do eat cheese, you buy dairy-free varieties.

Seeing on paper what you currently eat also may trigger the recognition of foods you're still eating that contain dairy. For instance, you may realize that you're using processed foods, such as cake mixes or salad dressings, that contain dairy ingredients. You may find that keeping a food diary helps you weed out the dairy products in stages, a batch at a time.

Do this every now and then so you stay aware of what you're eating. Maintaining a food diary not only documents what you're eating, but the very act of keeping the diary can make you change your behavior. If you've begun to slide a little, seeing what you've eaten can motivate you to be more vigilant in the future.

Getting help if you need it

If you find yourself stuck at some point along the way in your transition to going dairy-free, get some support. You have several options, including the following:

- ✔ **Get individualized diet counseling from a registered nutritionist.** A nutritionist can help you troubleshoot challenges and tailor advice for your specific concerns and lifestyle needs. In Chapter 4, I provide information about an online referral service you can use through the American Dietetic Association. This service helps you locate a dietitian in your area who can work with you.

  Check with your health insurance company to determine whether the cost of nutrition counseling may be covered in your case. If you have certain medical conditions, such as diabetes, coronary artery disease, or kidney problems, nutrition counseling services may be reimbursable if your physician refers you.

- ✔ **Talk to others going through the transition to a dairy-free diet.** You can ask them for advice on how they worked through challenges and stuck to their plans.

  One online resource is my blog, On the Table, where you can find links to other good resources as well as ongoing discussions about nutrition issues such as this one. To visit my blog, go to `www.onthetable.net`. You also can visit On the Table on Facebook.

- ✔ **Check other resources, including organizations and societies, books, and cookbooks.** All these resources can help you come up with additional dairy-free alternatives and meals, and can answer questions you may have. I include a list you can reference in the later sidebar "Accessing additional resources to keep you updated."

Making Sure Foods Are Dairy-Free

In order to successfully avoid dairy products, make sure you have the appropriate sleuthing skills and information sources. Being well informed includes having a good understanding of what to look for and how to read food labels.

It also means being savvy about changes that may occur from time to time in product formulas and getting the information you may need about these products from food companies. This section helps you get a better grasp of what's in products to help you ensure they're dairy-free.

Reading ingredient labels

If you're sensitive to dairy ingredients for any reason, you want to stay vigilant and bring all your good detective skills to bear when you decide what to eat. Not only do you have to look for the obvious sources of dairy, but you also have to catch the presence of even minor sources. The first place you can determine whether a food is dairy-free is on the product's ingredient label. Food labels are required to note all the ingredients included in a product during manufacturing.

In general, where food labels are concerned, short is good. That's because foods with short ingredient lists tend to be foods that are less processed and closer to their natural states. In other words, they tend to have fewer additives and byproducts that may be derivatives of dairy. Usually, though not always, a short ingredient list also means that figuring out what's inside the package is easier.

When you pick up a food product and read its label, pay attention to these issues, too:

✔ **Order of the ingredients:** Foods are listed in order of their predominance in the product. The ingredients listed first are present in the largest proportions in that product. Foods listed near the end are present in smaller quantities.

Knowing the order of the ingredients may help you decide whether you want to eat a particular food. You may not want to eat a food in which a dairy product is the first ingredient, but you may not mind it if that ingredient is at the tail end of the list. For example, if skim milk is listed first, you know that of the predominant ingredient in that product is milk. But if skim milk is listed last in a long line of ingredients, it's likely present in a very small amount. Depending on your reasons for living dairy-free, it may be okay for you to eat the product.

✔ **Potential allergens:** Since Congress passed the Food Allergen Labeling and Consumer Protection Act of 2004, ingredients for which the source is a major food allergen must be clearly identified on the food label.

Milk is one of the eight most common food allergens (the others are eggs, fish, shellfish, tree nuts, peanuts, wheat, and soybeans). So anything derived from milk has to be clearly labeled.

Here's how the law affects what you see on food labels. The dairy ingredient must be identified in one of two possible ways:

- ✔ **In parentheses following the name of the ingredient:** For example, whey may be listed on the label as "... whey (milk) ...." Similarly, casein may be listed as "... casein (milk) ...."

- ✔ **Immediately following or alongside the ingredient in a special statement that includes the word "contains":** For example, after an ingredient list on a food package, you may see the words, "Contains milk and soy." Another version you may see is, "May contain one or more of the following: milk, soy, or wheat."

You also may see wording on labels that indicates the potential for unintentional cross-contamination of foods with allergens. For example, a product processed on equipment that at times is used to process foods containing a food allergen may include on the label wording such as "Made on equipment that is also used to produce dairy beverages."

Be aware that foods labeled before January 1, 2006, weren't required to comply with the 2004 law and aren't required to have replacement labels. It's possible that some old food may be lingering on shelves in your home or in stores. If those products contain milk or milk byproducts, it may not be readily apparent to you by a quick scan of the ingredient list. So, if you're particularly sensitive or strict with your diet, take care to read food labels carefully in this type of situation.

If you can't read the labels of a food product and can't quite determine whether a dish has dairy in it, apply a healthy dose of caution to your food choices. This advice is especially wise if you're eating away from home and don't have a menu or product ingredient label to guide you. Wait staff at restaurants sometimes make mistakes or may not know that the creamy stuff inside the pasta is actually melted cheese. So let common sense be your guide. If you're not sure, assume it contains dairy. Check out Chapters 15 and 16 for advice on eating in social settings when you're not sure of the ingredients in food.

Communicating with food companies

In some cases, if a food's label doesn't give you the information you need (or you have further questions), you may be able to get the details about food ingredients directly from the horse's mouth — in this case the food companies. You can check a company's Web site, call a food manufacturer's customer service representative, or even put your question in writing and submit it to the company via e-mail or a written letter.

Accessing additional resources to keep you updated

Besides this great book you're currently reading, plenty of other good literary resources are available to help you work toward living dairy-free. Here are a few of my favorites:

✔ *Food Allergy Survival Guide* by **Vesanto Melina, Jo Stepaniak, and Dina Aronson (Healthy Living Publications):** This book covers practical information for understanding a range of food allergies and sensitivities, including dairy and other common problem foods.

✔ *The Ultimate Uncheese Cookbook* by **Joanne Stepaniak (Book Publishing Company):** This is an oldie but goodie. This skinny paperback cookbook includes a collection of creative recipes for making nondairy variations of common dairy-filled foods.

Many of the resources you'll find valuable for living dairy-free happen to be targeted at vegetarians and especially *vegans* (vegetarians who include no dairy foods in their diets). You'll find plenty of help from these vegetarian and vegan resources:

✔ **The Vegetarian Resource Group:** The Vegetarian Resource Group (VRG) is a U.S. nonprofit organization that educates the public about the interrelated issues of health, nutrition, ecology, ethics, and world hunger. The group publishes the bimonthly *Vegetarian Journal* and provides numerous other printed materials for consumers and health professionals. Most of the recipes and nutrition information come from the perspective of living dairy-free. The VRG health and nutrition materials are peer reviewed by registered dietitians and physicians. VRG also advocates for progressive changes in U.S. food and nutrition policy.

Reach VRG at P.O. Box 1463, Baltimore, MD 21203; phone 410-366-8343; fax 410-366-8803; e-mail vrg@vrg.org; Web site www.vrg.org. From the VRG Web site you can download and order materials, including handouts, reprints of articles, recipes, and more.

✔ **North American Vegetarian Society:** The North American Vegetarian Society (NAVS) is best known for its annual vegetarian conference, Summerfest, which often is held in Johnstown, Pennsylvania, in July. This casual, family-oriented conference draws an international crowd of 400 to 600 people each year. Nonvegetarians are welcome. Summerfest is an excellent opportunity to sample fabulous dairy-free foods, meet others who are interested in eating fewer animal products, attend lectures, and pick up materials from a variety of vegetarian organizations, most of which promote a diet that's dairy-free. The group publishes *The Vegetarian Voice,* a newsletter for members.

You can contact NAVS at P.O. Box 72, Dolgeville, NY 13329; phone 518-568-7970; e-mail navs@telenet.net; Web site www.navs-online.org.

✔ **The Physicians Committee for Responsible Medicine:** The Physicians Committee for Responsible Medicine (PCRM) is a nonprofit organization of physicians and others who work together to advocate for compassionate and effective medical practices, research, and health promotion, including dairy-free and vegetarian diets. The PCRM publishes the quarterly newsletter *Good Medicine.*

You can contact PCRM at 5100 Wisconsin Ave., NW, Suite 400, Washington, DC 20016; phone 202-686-2210; fax 202-686-2216; e-mail `pcrm@pcrm.org`; Web site `www.pcrm.org`.

✔ **The Vegetarian Nutrition Dietetic Practice Group:** The Vegetarian Nutrition Dietetic Practice Group (VNDPG) is a subgroup within the American Dietetic Association (ADA) for dietitians with a special interest in vegetarian diets, including those that are dairy-free. The group publishes a quarterly newsletter, and other consumer nutrition education materials are available online at `www.vegetariannutrition.net`.

The ADA also offers a referral service for people who need individual nutrition counseling. To find the name and contact information of a registered dietitian in your area with expertise in vegetarian or dairy-free diets, visit `www.eatright.org`.

Listen to that little voice in your head; if you sense that the person at the other end of the telephone isn't confident about his response to your question, don't take his word for it. Ask to speak with a supervisor, or call back another day and speak with someone else. And double-check any response you get by calling back and asking someone else or cross-checking information on the company's Web site. Customer service representatives have been known to make mistakes.

Customers who have been misled or misinformed about product ingredients have sued food companies. For this reason, companies usually take consumer inquiries about food ingredients seriously. With a little persistence, you should be able to get an answer to your question about food ingredients.

Focusing on Some Detailed Dairy-Free Advice

Good for you for taking these first steps to living dairy-free! You're on your way, and you're going to be fine. If you had any doubts about whether you could still enjoy food and get along with your family and friends without including dairy products in your diet, those concerns should be melting away like an ice cream cone on a hot summer day. After you have a basic foundation for going dairy-free, you may be ready for more in-depth advice, which I give you in this section.

Surveying supermarkets for alternatives

When you decide to remove the dairy from your diet, the first step is identifying all the dairy products you commonly eat and taking them off your shopping list. The next step, though, can be the real stumper. After all, figuring out what you *can* eat in place of those foods you remove from your diet can be tricky.

If you like to shop, you'll love this step. One of the best ways to get familiar with the dairy-free choices you have is to peruse a variety of supermarkets for nondairy alternatives. I go into much more detail in Chapters 6 and 7 about different types of stores you should visit as well as the specific products to try.

For now, keep a few points in mind as you get ready to move on:

- ✔ **Special products aren't required.** Living dairy-free doesn't require you to spend a lot of money buying dairy substitutes and other specialty products. You don't have to replace everything. Just because you give up mozzarella cheese, for example, doesn't mean you need to replace it with a soy-based alternative. Many people do very well without eating any form of cheese whatsoever, thank-you-very-much.

   If you want to use nondairy substitutes for dairy products such as milk, cheese, yogurt, sour cream, and ice cream, that's fine. Just realize upfront that they're optional.

- ✔ **Take the opportunity to explore.** Be free! Venture into some stores and experiment with some products you've never tried before. It's your chance to get creative and break out of old ways of doing things.

- ✔ **Accept some conveniences.** The healthiest foods around are those in their simplest, natural forms — fresh fruits, vegetables, and whole grains, for example. Even though these foods are the best, we don't always want to fix everything we eat from scratch. At times — maybe more often than not — you have to rely on convenience foods that make it quicker to put a meal on the table. Convenience foods are okay, and they add variety to your diet, too.

   So, for example, recognize that when you spread nondairy cream cheese on your bagel or sprinkle shredded, mozzarella-style nondairy cheese on your pizza, you're eating processed foods. That's okay. As long as you also include plenty of unprocessed foods in your diet, a few convenience products can be enjoyable additions to a healthy, dairy-free diet.

- ✔ **Count on some duds.** When you experiment with new, dairy-free products that you find at the supermarket, you'll like some and be disappointed with others. That's just the way it goes. In this book, I try to steer you to some of the products I've tried and think are best. But you have to be the ultimate judge of what's good and not good for *you.* What you and I like and expect from foods differs.

Explaining your diet to family and friends

You may make the personal decision to go dairy-free based on several reasons — and you may not spread the news right away. However, after you stick with your plan for a while and feel more confident and comfortable with your lifestyle change, you may have to talk about it with your friends and family. For some people, doing so may be no big deal, but for others, it may be more difficult.

The good news: Getting along on a diet that's outside the norm is easier than ever. Consider the following reasons:

- ✔ Increasingly more people are aware of food intolerances or have political convictions that influence what they do and don't eat.
- ✔ You can find more specialty food available in supermarkets.
- ✔ As the country's population becomes more diverse with newcomers from different parts of the world, more ethnic markets and restaurants are opening Americans' eyes and taste buds to new foods from around the world.

For all these reasons, you're likely to find that telling friends and family about a change in your eating style isn't difficult. When you do, they're likely to understand.

However, if you do have a difficult time explaining your dairy-free lifestyle to family and friends, Chapter 15 provides helpful tips, including what to say to people who may be curious about your food choices.

Anticipating meals outside your home

As you make the move to living dairy-free, it's natural that your initial focus will be on what to eat and what to avoid. Very quickly, though, you'll find that you also need to give some attention to various social situations you encounter. Food, after all, plays a major role in most people's social lives. For that reason, expect that you'll have some adjustments to make when you eat meals away from home.

You need to think about the following issues:

- ✔ **Eating at other people's homes:** When you're a guest at someone else's house, you need to warn them about your food preferences before you arrive for dinner. If you don't, you need a strategy for making do with whatever is served — without offending your host! I cover this topic in detail in Chapter 15, including lots of tips and strategies for dealing with a variety of situations in which you want to be a gracious guest.

✔ **Getting what you need at restaurants:** Because dairy products are so widespread throughout the standard American diet, you'll find them worked (often sneakily) into soups, salads, entrees, sides, breads, and desserts. So successfully dodging dairy when you go out to eat requires you to exercise some special skills. You need to read menus carefully, be assertive and ask questions of your wait staff, and be creative about suggesting workarounds. I include lots of good ideas for doing this in Chapter 16.

✔ **Keeping kids healthy and well fed at school:** If you have a child who needs to avoid dairy products, she likely requires help getting what she needs — and avoiding what she doesn't need — at school. School staff and food service personnel may be helpful in suggesting suitable alternatives and strategies for feeding your child while she's at school. In fact, it's becoming much more common for schools to provide some children with alternatives to cow's milk with their meals. *Remember:* Schools may require you to bring in a doctor's note in order for them to provide your child with fortified soymilk or other alternatives.

It's important to talk with your child about what her choices are at school. You may want to get a copy of the menu ahead of time, review it with your child, and discuss what she'll choose when she gets to the lunch line. I provide more information about helping your child manage school meals in Chapter 18.

Setting realistic expectations

As you're transitioning to a dairy-free diet, remember to set practical and realistic expectations for your progress. And be sure to anticipate that you may have a setback now and then. If you do, it's not the end of the world. At your next meal, focus on getting back on track.

Don't be too hard on yourself. Any lifestyle change is difficult to make. It's especially difficult for adults who have to relearn a lifetime of eating habits. You didn't develop your current eating style overnight. It will take more than an overnight effort to feel comfortable with something new.

Also keep in mind that you'll encounter vacations, holidays, and sick days. You'll find yourself in social situations where you may go with the flow — even if it includes dairy — just for old time's sake. All these situations are times in which you may have a momentary lapse and down a cheese cracker or bowl of cream of potato soup. When these times come (and they will), take them in stride. Just pick up where you left off, and move on. You need to be flexible enough to allow yourself some wiggle room. Slowly but surely the lapses will happen less frequently as you acquire the skills and confidence you need to stick with your new eating style.

Part II
Setting Up Your Dairy-Free Kitchen

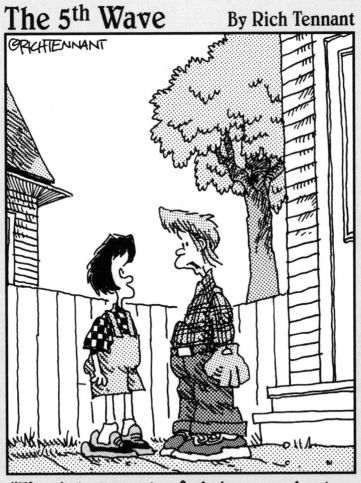

The 5th Wave   By Rich Tennant

"I'm intolerant of dairy products, and I'm barely getting along with spinach and beets."

In this part . . .

There's no place like home for nutritious, good-tasting, dairy-free meals. That's why this part of the book is dedicated to helping you gather the ingredients, tools, and skills you need to turn meal ideas into plates full of home-cooked goodness.

I start by helping you identify and remove the dairy products stashed in the refrigerator, freezer, and pantry. From there, I offer some suggestions for versatile, nondairy replacements. Next, I cover what you need to know about where to shop for nondairy staples and strategies for getting the best values. I round out this part with a chapter on practical equipment and basic cooking techniques.

Chapter 6

Removing Dairy from Your Kitchen

In This Chapter

▶ Figuring out which foods contain dairy and purging them

▶ Swapping dairy with nondairy ingredients

▶ Understanding the unique features of nondairy alternatives

So you've made the decision to go dairy-free. Now it's time to conduct a thorough search of your kitchen to find the dairy products and dairy byproducts stored in your pantry, refrigerator, and cupboards. With this information in hand, you can remove the unwanted foods and replace many of them with versatile, good-tasting substitutes that are widely available today. In fact, you may be surprised to find out how many choices you have.

In this chapter, I help you identify the main dairy culprits in your kitchen so you can discard them or give them to friends and family. I then describe practical dairy-free substitutes for common dairy products. You may have heard of some of them, and you even may have tried a few. But others will likely be unfamiliar to you. All are healthful, multipurpose products worth knowing about and keeping on hand. I also explain some of the special features common to nondairy products that you need to know about to help you make well-informed choices when you shop.

Uncovering Dairy Items in Your Kitchen and Tossing Them

In order to get rid of dairy products in your home, keep this fun phrase in mind: Seek and sweep them out. *Translation:* You want to locate the dairy items and remove them.

You don't have to be wasteful and throw the foods away. Pass them on to others who can use them, such as your neighbors or co-workers. But whatever you do with them, remove these products from the active inventory of supplies in your own kitchen.

In this section, I help you identify the foods you need to replace in order to go dairy-free. Some may be obvious to you, but others take more work to single out. Read food labels carefully to be sure you're catching all the dairy-containing foods you need to find. If you need more help, Chapter 5 contains label-reading advice and tips for spotting hidden sources of dairy.

The big three: Milk, cheese, and yogurt

If you're like most people, cow's milk, various kinds of cheese, and yogurt are the major dairy products in your home. If you want to go totally dairy-free, you need to remove all these foods from your home. They come in many varieties. Look for the following:

- ✔ **Cow's milk:** Whole, low-fat (2 percent, 1 percent, ½ percent), skim, buttermilk, eggnog, and flavored milk (such as chocolate and strawberry)

- ✔ **Cheese:** Cheddar, cottage, farmer, havarti, jack, mozzarella, Muenster, Parmesan, provolone, ricotta, Swiss, cream cheese, and others

- ✔ **Yogurt:** Regular, low-fat, nonfat, flavored, plain, and *kefir* (a fermented drink made from cow's milk)

Kefir can be pronounced correctly as ke-fir, ke-feer, or kee-fir. Kefir sold in North America usually is made from cow's milk, but it also can be made using sheep or goat milk. Milk from sheep and goats can cause the same problems for people that cow's milk causes.

Most dairy products sold in North America are made with cow's milk, but milk from other mammals, including goats, sheep, and water buffaloes, also is used in many parts of the world. Some of these dairy products are imported and sold in North America. For example, Greek-style or salad cheese usually is made from any combination of milk from cows, goats, or sheep. Authentic *feta* cheese, a pungent, white, crumbly cheese from Greece, is made from the milk of special breeds of sheep and goats.

When you peruse your kitchen for milk, cheese, and yogurt, remember to check packaged foods. You may find frozen entrees such as lasagna, dry mixes such as macaroni and cheese, and yogurt-covered granola or cereal bars that contain dairy foods as primary or minor ingredients.

As you remove the milk, cheese, and yogurt products from your kitchen, understand that the fat, protein, and carbohydrate (including lactose) contents may vary greatly, depending on specific factors such as the type of milk used. These content levels may be relevant to you, depending on your reasons for limiting dairy products or the extent to which you opt to avoid certain products.

For example, a 2-ounce chunk of full-fat, extra-sharp cheddar cheese contains at least 10 grams of artery-clogging saturated fat. The same amount of 2-percent-fat cheddar cheese contains about half as much saturated fat. If you're limiting dairy products to reduce your risk for coronary artery disease, you may decide to completely rid your house of full-fat cheese but keep a small amount of reduced-fat cheese to use on occasion.

However, in general, milk, cheese, and yogurt are substantial sources of lactose, milk protein, and, with the exception of fat-free varieties, saturated fat. All are fiberless. (In Chapter 3, I provide a comparison of the levels of lactose in various types of dairy foods, because some people with lactose intolerance may be able to tolerate small amounts of foods that are very low in lactose.)

Spreads: Butter and margarine

To maintain a dairy-free kitchen, you need to eliminate spreads. *Spreads* are products like butter that you can cover something else with, like a piece of bread. The following are the main types of spreads to watch out for:

✔ **Butter:** This spread usually is made from cow's milk, but in some parts of the world, it's sometimes made from the milk of other animals. The lactose content of butter is relatively low and may not bother some people with lactose intolerance. Butter is high in saturated fat, though, and it also contains milk proteins.

✔ **Blended spreads:** These products are made with dairy butter that has been mixed with vegetable oils, such as canola oil or olive oil to make a soft spread. These products generally are healthier choices than all-butter spreads, but they may still contain more saturated fat or lactose than you care to eat.

✔ **Margarine:** This type of spread is made primarily with vegetable oils. The oils often are *partially hydrogenated,* a form of processing that adds hydrogen to liquid oils and hardens them. Partially hydrogenated oil may be soft (as in tub margarine) or firm enough to hold the shape of a stick, depending on how much hydrogen has been added. So you'll find margarine sold in sticks, tubs, and squeeze bottles.

Partially hydrogenated oils contain *trans fats,* which, like saturated fats, are associated with increased risk for coronary artery disease. So margarine spreads that contain trans fats carry the same health risks as those dairy sources that are rich in saturated fat. The best forms of dairy-free margarine are also trans-fat-free.

Be sure to read package labels carefully to determine whether various brands of butter, margarine, and blended spreads contain dairy ingredients. Manufacturers frequently introduce new products into stores, and even existing products can undergo formula changes. By spot-checking labels from time to time, you may catch changes that you need to know about.

Toppers: Sour cream and whipped cream

You also want to get rid of the dairy toppers that you add to food to give it a creamy taste. The culprits include the following:

- **Cream:** It's the butterfat layer skimmed from cow's milk. It's rich in saturated fat and also contains small amounts of lactose and milk proteins.

- **Half-n-half:** It's the half-cream-and-half-milk product for coffee drinkers. Some people like it on their oatmeal or strawberries, too.

- **Sour cream:** It's cream that has been soured using a bacterial culture. People use sour cream in baking, to make sauces, or to top baked potatoes, blintzes, potato pancakes, or burritos.

- **Whipped cream:** It's made by whisking or whipping air into cream that has a high butterfat content. If you don't whip your own cream by hand or with an electric mixer, you probably buy it ready-to-use in a can. These commercial products use nitrous oxide to whip the cream as it comes out of the spray can.

- **Miscellaneous products:** Other dairy toppers you may see include the following:

    - French *crème fraîche* and Mexican *crema* or *cream espresa* are similar to sour cream but not as sour or thick.

    - *Clotted cream,* which is popular in the United Kingdom, is cream that has been thickened through a drying process. It's often served as a topper or spread on baked goods such as scones.

    - Very thick variations of sour cream are used around the world in cooking and as an accompaniment with foods. Examples include *Smetana* (Central and Eastern Europe), *rjome* or *romme* (Norway), and *rjomi* (Iceland).

Cool Whip, a popular imitation whipped cream or topping, is often thought to be nondairy because it contains no milk or cream and is lactose-free. However, it does contain sodium caseinate, a dairy byproduct made from the milk protein casein.

The sweets: Ice cream and dairy desserts

Check your freezer for ice cream and other frozen desserts made from milk, cream, and other dairy ingredients. Examples include the following:

- ✔ Premium, low-fat, and nonfat brands of ice cream
- ✔ Sherbet and sorbets made with milk (check labels)
- ✔ Ice cream sandwiches, bars, cups, and other frozen novelties
- ✔ Cakes, pies, tortes, cream puffs, and similar desserts filled with ice cream, cream, and other dairy ingredients

Check your pantry and cupboards, too, for canned or packaged desserts and mixes that may contain powdered milk, cheese, cream, and other dairy ingredients. Examples include pudding mixes and pie fillings as well as cookie, bar, and other dessert mixes.

Other minor sources

You may find it easy to spot the obvious sources of dairy in your home — a half gallon of milk, a carton of ice cream, and a block of cheese. However, you also want to keep an eye open for other foods that may have some dairy ingredients in them. Dairy products are added to many processed foods, even if only in small amounts.

Read the ingredient labels on food packages carefully to identify hidden sources of dairy products. I include a list of frequently used and often hard-to-spot dairy byproducts in Chapter 5.

Replacing Dairy with Nondairy Alternatives

Almost every dairy product you can name has a nondairy counterpart that tastes great and can be used in the same ways. You've probably seen many of these products while walking down your grocery store's aisles. For example, milk replacers such as soy, almond, and rice milks are sold in many mainstream supermarkets and natural foods stores. Soy-based coffee creamers are easy to find, too. Many other options are available for you to replace your dairy foods, and in the following sections, I describe what's available. (Chapter 21 provides some more information on many of the products you read about here.)

Introducing nondairy milk, cheese, and yogurt

Get ready to be pleasantly surprised if you've never tried these replacement products for your milk, cheese, and yogurt. Most of them are delicious and, with a few exceptions, they work well as replacements for their dairy counterparts.

Nondairy milk

Nondairy varieties of milk are the stars of dairy-free eating. That's because these products taste so good. You can use these nondairy milk products in the same ways you use cow's milk in cooking and baking and on your breakfast cereal or with a plate of cookies. Even better: All these nondairy milks are lactose-free and don't have the saturated fats that cow's milk does.

A slight downside: You'll probably notice the difference in flavor and appearance between nondairy milk and cow's milk when you first try these products. Each form of nondairy milk has its own unique flavor and consistency, and none tastes or looks exactly like cow's milk. However, most of these milk replacers taste really good, and you're sure to find a favorite or two. Soymilk has a mild, beany flavor, while almond milk and rice milk each have a mild, pleasant flavor. Or, if you prefer, buy your milk replacers flavored with almond, vanilla, chocolate, or carob.

I have used these products for many years, and I have spoken with many people who also have made the switch. You may have a preference for a particular type of nondairy milk or a specific brand, but I'm confident that you'll find a product you like.

Oh soy! Understanding the pros and cons

From time to time, reports surface in the media concerning links between soy foods and various health risks, including breast cancer and thyroid disease in adults and immune system in babies. In general, though, no convincing evidence exists that soy foods such as soymilk, soy-based ice cream, or soy yogurt pose any health risks.

On the contrary, these foods tend to offer health advantages when they replace dairy-based products in the diet. Two-thirds of the fat in dairy products are artery-clogging saturated fat. Replacing fatty dairy products, such as cheese, yogurt, and milk, with soy-based products can lower your intake of saturated fat as well as your risk for coronary artery disease.

One caveat needs to be noted, however. Some people are allergic to soy protein. If you're allergic to soy, use almond or rice milk products instead.

The most common and popular varieties include

- **Soymilk:** This nondairy milk is made from soaked, ground, and strained soybeans. Buy it plain, or try the vanilla-, chocolate-, or carob-flavored varieties. During the holidays, you also may find soy-based eggnog. Soymilk has a mild flavor.

  Some supermarkets, warehouse stores such as Costco, and specialty stores such as Trader Joe's, carry their own private-label soymilk. Other popular brands include Silk, EdenSoy, Organic Valley, Pacific, Vitasoy, Westsoy, and others.

- **Rice milk:** This grain milk usually is made with brown rice. It's thinner in consistency than soymilk and whiter in color. It resembles cow's milk in appearance more than other forms of nondairy milk. Rice milk has a mild flavor. Buy it plain, or try the vanilla-, carob-, or chocolate-flavored varieties.

  Rice milk is the nondairy beverage tolerated best by the most people. That's because rice is one of the most hypoallergenic foods. Rice milk is tolerated well by people who are lactose intolerant and those who have soy or tree-nut allergies. In general, though, it's less nutritious than soymilk, which contains more protein and calcium.

  Rice Dream is a popular brand that's easy to find in many mainstream supermarkets. Trader Joe's has its own private-label rice milk as well.

- **Almond milk:** Blend finely ground nuts with water, and you have almond milk. It has a mild, nutty flavor with a rich consistency similar to that of soymilk. Like soymilk and rice milk, almond milk is sold in a few different flavors. Brands you'll commonly find in mainstream supermarkets and natural foods stores include Almond Breeze and Almond Dream.

  Like rice milk, almond milk is a nondairy option for people who are allergic to soy. It contains less protein than soymilk, but fortified almond milk is comparable to fortified soymilk in calcium, vitamin D, and other vitamins and minerals (though it may not be fortified with vitamin B12). People who are allergic to tree nuts may have to avoid almond milk, though.

- **Other forms of nondairy milk:** Natural foods stores also carry less familiar forms of milk, including nondairy milks made from oats and potatoes. These aren't as popular, nor are they as widely available, as other nondairy milks. But they may be useful for people who, for whatever reason, don't care for or can't use soy, rice, or almond milks.

Most brands of soymilk, almond milk, and rice milk are fortified or enriched with calcium and vitamins A and D. This fortification generally brings them in line with the nutritional content of cow's milk. Though keep in mind that rice milk is lower in protein. Also keep in mind that none of these nondairy milks are suitable replacements for infant formula.

Nondairy cheese

Most cheese substitutes are made from soy, though some also are made from rice milk, almond milk, and other nondairy ingredients. Experiment with different brands — and different varieties within brands — to find those you like the best. The flavors and textures of nondairy cheeses vary a lot.

Be aware that many cheese substitutes, including many made mostly from soy, rice, and other nondairy ingredients, contain small amounts of dairy byproducts such as casein. Read ingredient labels to be sure. Review the information in Chapter 5 to make yourself aware of hidden dairy byproducts that may be present in these foods.

Cheese substitutes are sold as bricks, in slices, and shredded. They come in many familiar cheese flavors, including mozzarella, pepper jack, American, cheddar, and others. You also can buy nondairy cream cheese–like products. Some widely available brands of cheese include Tofutti, TofuRella, Galaxy Nutritional Foods, and Lifetime. You'll find the largest selection in natural foods stores.

A good-tasting substitute for Parmesan cheese is *nutritional yeast.* Nutritional yeast is a savory, nutty, rich-tasting variety of yeast sold in flakes or as a yellow powder in natural foods stores.

Nondairy yogurt

Soy-based, nondairy yogurt products are available in many mainstream supermarkets and most natural foods stores. The consistency of nondairy yogurts is often thinner or looser when compared to yogurt made from cow's milk. The flavor is generally excellent. They're available in many flavors as well as plain or fruited. Two examples of popular, good-tasting brands include Silk Live! and WholeSoy yogurt.

Nondairy milk, yogurt, ice cream, and other products made with coconut milk also are available in some stores. These products have many benefits, because they're dairy-free and also work for people who may be allergic to soy or almonds. They taste great, are rich in calcium, and may be fortified with vitamin B12, an important addition for strict vegetarians or vegans who need a reliable source of this important nutrient. On the other hand, these products are high in saturated fat from the coconut milk, so they may increase the risk of coronary artery disease by stimulating your body to make more cholesterol.

Bringing in nondairy spreads and toppings

You can find dozens of varieties of butter substitutes and margarines in supermarkets, but you need to read labels carefully to find those that contain no dairy byproducts. Review the information in Chapter 5 to become familiar with the range of dairy byproducts that often are added in small amounts to many processed foods.

Look for butter and margarine products that are labeled *pareve* or *parve.* You can be sure that these foods contain no dairy ingredients. Pareve or parve (PAR-uh-vuh or PAR-vuh) is a designation in Jewish dietary law that means the food contains no dairy or meat byproducts. People who keep *kosher,* or adhere to Jewish dietary laws, don't eat meat and dairy ingredients at the same meal. Foods that are pareve are neutral and can be eaten at any meal containing meat or dairy foods. Examples of products that are pareve include Fleishmann's Light Margarine, Smart Balance Light, and Earth Balance tub margarines, among others.

If you're severely allergic to dairy products, however, be careful. Even kosher foods may be contaminated with tiny particles of dairy from food production lines that may be adjacent to those that are processing foods labeled as pareve or parve. Tiny particles of dairy may be able to migrate through the air and land in products that are otherwise dairy-free. The chances are slim, but it's possible.

Adding nondairy ice cream and frozen desserts

You can find a variety of delicious ice cream substitutes and frozen novelties made with nondairy ingredients in natural foods stores and some mainstream supermarkets. Look for varieties made from soy, rice, nuts, fruit juices, and other nondairy ingredients. Some of these products, such as those made by Rice Dream, Tofutti, and other popular brands, are similar in flavor and consistency to ice cream. Others are more like fruit sorbet. Dole and Nouvelle Sorbet are two popular examples.

A limited number of cakes, pies, tortes, and other desserts made with nondairy ingredients are available in the frozen foods case. Read ingredient labels carefully (and review Chapter 5 for discussion about hidden sources of dairy ingredients in packaged foods).

Rating the best for taste and function

People have different opinions about which dairy-free products are best, mainly because you have so many products to choose from and so many factors to consider. When deciding your own favorites, you have to keep both of the following in mind:

✔ **Taste:** Your tastes obviously are going to differ from the next person's. For example, some people prefer the thin consistency and neutral flavor of rice milk. Others find the creamier, mild flavor of soymilk to be quite delicious. Even within types of products, opinions differ. I personally like Silk soymilk the best (EdenSoy is a close runner-up). Silk tastes great, and it doesn't curdle when I add it to my coffee like some other brands do. I also like Rice Dream rice milk and Almond Breeze almond milk.

You, however, may come to entirely different conclusions. Experiment with different products to find those you think taste best. Your preferences also may change over time. For instance, many people don't care for the flavor of soymilk the first time they try it. Later, it grows on them, and they end up loving it.

✔ **Function:** Similarly, your experience with the function of different products may vary, depending on how you use them. Cheese substitutes may work well blended into a casserole where they can melt thoroughly and mix with other ingredients. Served in chunks with crackers or sliced onto a sandwich, though, they may seem rubbery in consistency or lack the creamy mouth feel of dairy cheese.

You may enjoy reading others' opinions about the products they've tried. Surf the Web for blog posts and reviews of products. (Blog sites change often, so I won't attempt to list them here; just use your browser to do a search for non-dairy milk, cheese, yogurt, or whatever product you're interested in.) Check blogs devoted to lactose intolerance or vegan diets. If you don't see comments that directly address your questions, post your own questions on the blog.

Whip up your own nut milk

Making your own nut milk is easy and fun. To make almond milk, just follow these easy steps:

1. **Soak one cup of whole almonds in water overnight.**

2. **Pour off the water from the soaked almonds, and then blanch them by dipping them into boiling water for 30 seconds or so.**

   Blanching the almonds helps the fibrous skins to come off. Use a stainless steel or other mesh strainer to dip almonds into the water and remove them easily.

3. **Rinse the nuts to remove the skins, and then grind the nuts finely in a food processor.**

4. **Add 4 cups of water (fresh water or feel free to recycle the water used to soak the almonds) and blend thoroughly and chill.**

   To remove flecks of dark nut matter, you can strain the milk through a coffee filter or cheesecloth.

The same process can be used to make any kind of nut milk. Experiment with cashews, walnuts, pecans, and others. To sweeten the milk slightly, add a teaspoon or two of honey, maple syrup, agave syrup, or rice syrup. You also can add a teaspoon or two of pure vanilla extract for additional flavor. Fresh nut milk keeps in the refrigerator for up to about two weeks.

Putting nondairy products to use

After you begin tasting and working with different nondairy products, you'll become more familiar and comfortable with incorporating them into your daily diet. You can discover which brands you and your family like best, and then you can experiment to find new ways to use them.

In Chapter 7, I include more information about where to shop for various nondairy products and how to determine which products you may find most useful. In Chapter 8, I provide lots of information about how to cook with nondairy ingredients, including ways to modify traditional recipes to make them dairy-free.

Pointing Out Some Special Features of Nondairy Alternatives

The nondairy products you can incorporate into your dairy-free kitchen are incredibly convenient and versatile. They share many of the same features as dairy products. For example, you can use any kind of nondairy milk cup for cup to replace cow's milk in a recipe. Furthermore, you can use most forms of nondairy cheese just like dairy cheese in recipes. However, I do point out some differences between dairy and nondairy products in this section.

Packaging is unique

One of the main differences between dairy and nondairy products is the packaging. Although most dairy milk packaging includes conventional containers that require refrigeration, many varieties of soymilk, almond milk, and rice milk are sold on grocery store shelves in *aseptic* cartons. Aseptic packaging permits foods to remain on store shelves or unopened in your cupboard at home for several months without refrigeration. However, once you open a carton, you must refrigerate it.

Some brands of nondairy milk are sold in two forms of packaging: in aseptic cartons as well as in conventional quart and half-gallon containers. Nondairy milk sold in conventional containers usually is sold alongside cow's milk in the refrigerator section of the grocery store. Packaging for other nondairy products — ice cream, spreads, and cheese — are generally the same as for the dairy varieties.

Looking at shelf life

Nondairy products such as milk, cheese, spreads, and frozen desserts have shelf lives similar to those of dairy products. The exception is nondairy milk in aseptic packaging. You can keep unopened nondairy milk in aseptic packaging in your cabinet for as long as a year before using it. Your best bet, though, is to look at the "use by" date marked on the package to be sure the product is still fresh when you use it.

If you store several containers of nondairy milk at the same time, rotate your stock so that you use older products before the newer ones.

After you open aseptic packages of nondairy milk, make sure you store the product in the fridge, just like regular cow's milk. After you open them, you can keep aseptic cartons of soymilk, almond milk, and rice milk for at least two weeks in the fridge before they begin to sour.

Chapter 7

Shopping for and Stocking Your Dairy-Free Home

- -

- -

After you remove from your kitchen the dairy products that you can't or don't want to eat (as I discuss in Chapter 6), you need to fill it with nondairy products you can and do want to eat. Doing so is easy if you have some strategies in mind to help you shop effectively. Stocking your home with good-tasting, versatile foods can help ensure that you have lots of quick and easy options at mealtimes.

My goal for this chapter is to help you understand what you need and where to go to find the most practical and essential food supplies. You're going to fill your kitchen with dairy-free staples. What are you waiting for? It's time to go shopping.

Determining What You Need by Planning Ahead

Having a plan before you set foot in the store is a smart move. If you plan ahead, you're more likely to have on hand a variety of ingredients for fixing nutritious meals that you and your family will love. You're less likely to forget critical ingredients, too. And when you plan ahead, you're less likely to come home with a bag full of things you don't need that you bought on impulse.

Eating dairy-free can be a completely healthful way to live, but you also want to make sure that whatever diet you eat is as health-supporting as it can be. After all, chips and soft drinks are dairy-free, but they don't make for a very healthful diet!

As you craft your shopping plan, think about your overall nutritional goals and needs. After you have a plan, you can draft your shopping list. In this section, I help you get started.

Mapping out meal plans

By planning out your meals before you go shopping, you allow yourself to eat more healthfully. That's because you can make sure you're getting all the nutrients you need at each meal with your dairy-free lifestyle. Planning your menu in advance also can save you time and money. After all, who wants to plan and shop for dinner after a hard days' work? Not many people. And, in this situation, many folks end up going out to eat for convenience's sake.

In Chapter 4, I explain dairy-free nutrition: How and where to get your calcium, vitamin D, and all the other essential nutrients you need on a diet without dairy products. How does all of this translate into a shopping plan? You can use that information to inspire yourself with regard to creating your shopping lists and planning your menus. To help you map your own meal plans, I cover two resources in the following sections.

MyPyramid

One tool you can use to create your own meal plans is the U.S. government's guide to eating right, called the MyPyramid. The MyPyramid graphic (check out Figure 7-1), which includes a stick figure walking up the side of the pyramid, represents the steps to eating well by depicting the roles of diet and exercise.

The main pyramid in the graphic is divided into smaller pyramids, with each section representing a grouping of foods you should choose. Detailed information about the foods in each group is included online at the MyPyramid Web site (www.mypyramid.gov/pyramid/index.html).

The site includes an interactive menu planner that can help you create an individualized meal plan. The site also includes information about how to adapt the plan if you're lactose intolerant.

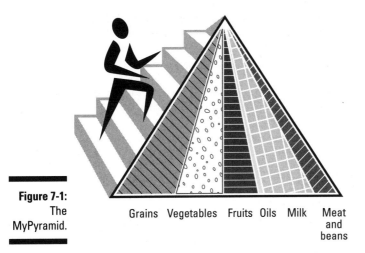

Figure 7-1:
The
MyPyramid.

Grains Vegetables Fruits Oils Milk Meat and beans

Food guide for North American vegetarians

A second meal planner I like may be more appropriate and easier to use for some readers. This guide (see Figure 7-2) was created for vegetarians who may not eat dairy products, so it clearly shows what the choices are for someone who doesn't drink milk or eat milk products. You can read more about it online at: www.dietitians.ca/news/downloads/Vegetarian_Food_Guide_for_NA.pdf.

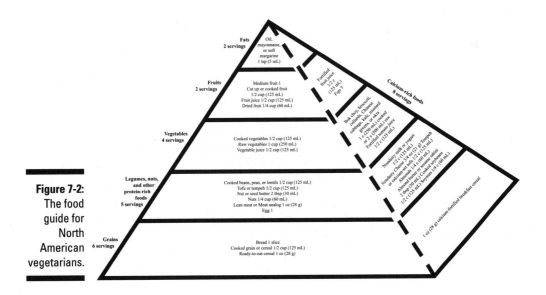

Figure 7-2:
The food
guide for
North
American
vegetarians.

You don't have to be a vegetarian to use this food guide (meat eaters can substitute meat where "protein-rich foods" are listed on the plan). If you use it, though, it helps to ensure that your diet includes the full range of nutrients you need, with special emphasis on calcium.

Whether you're a vegetarian or a meat eater, if you use Figure 7-2 to guide your meal planning, keep the following advice in mind:

- **Make variety the spice of your life.** Eat a variety of foods, and get enough servings of each food group to meet your calorie needs.

- **Get your calcium.** Eat at least eight servings of calcium-rich foods from the vegetarian food guide. These can count as servings from other food groups at the same time. For example, a serving of calcium-fortified orange juice also can be counted as a serving from the fruit group.

- **Count nuts and seeds as servings from the fat group.** That's because nuts and seeds get most of their calories from fat.

- **Make sure your vitamin D intake is sufficient.** Get enough vitamin D through sun exposure, eating fortified foods, or taking a supplement.

- **Aim for more vitamin B12.** If you're a vegetarian, you should get at least three reliable food sources of vitamin B12 in your diet every day. One serving is equal to any of the following:

  - 1 tablespoon of Red Star Vegetarian Support Formula nutritional yeast

  - 1 cup fortified soymilk or other fortified nondairy milk

  - 1 ounce of fortified breakfast cereal

  If you don't consistently get enough vitamin B12 from food sources, take a B12 supplement. Aim for 5–10 μg each day or take a weekly supplement of 2,000 μg. (If you're a nonvegetarian, you don't have to worry about B12, because you can get enough from meat, fish, poultry, and eggs.)

- **Watch those empty calories.** Keep your intake of sweets and alcohol to a minimum to help ensure that you have enough room in your diet for the nutritious foods listed in the food guide.

Keeping a grocery list

Maintaining a grocery list of the items you need is an important process of shopping. In fact, I'm a big fan of keeping a grocery list. A grocery list can help you stay organized. If you maintain a running list of what you need — and add to it whenever you notice you're running low on something — you stand a much better chance of coming home with that food when you shop. A grocery list also can help you curb the impulse to buy things you shouldn't eat or don't need. The list helps you focus and not get distracted by other items on the store shelves.

How you use your grocery list is up to you. Some people like to plan a week's worth of meals at a time, and they shop for those supplies once a week. Other people — including me — prefer to keep a supply of staples on hand at all times. When my family runs low on different items, we add them to our list. We may shop for perishable foods — fruits, vegetables, deli items, and refrigerated cartons of almond milk, for example — once a week. But we shop for cupboard supplies — pasta, cereal, and rice milk in aseptic cartons — about once a month.

Less-experienced cooks — and people who like to know in advance what they're having for dinner each night — often like the structure of planning meals on a weekly basis. Other people like the flexibility of keeping things looser. When it's time to make a meal at our house, my family and I see what we feel like making at the moment and then draw from the ingredients we have on hand. When putting together your own list, do what's right for you.

The grocery lists I include in the following sections aren't comprehensive. They're just some nondairy examples to help you get started. You want to round out these lists with your favorite staples, including any fruits, vegetables, bread and cereal products, and other foods you need to plan a variety of meals you enjoy making. I include on these lists a wide range of nondairy foods and other products that I find particularly useful for people who don't eat dairy products. You may not want or need all the items on these lists. They're simply included as suggestions. I organize the items in two categories: those you likely need to buy weekly (because they don't stay fresh very long) and those you can buy less often. You can read about many of the nondairy items I list in Chapter 6.

Consider typing and printing a list of foods that you use on a regular basis and buy often. Keep a copy in a convenient spot, and circle or mark the foods you need before your next shopping trip. Seeing the items pre-listed may help you remember to buy items that you're low on. And be sure to keep your list in a place that's easy to see when you want to add to it. The refrigerator door, a desk in the kitchen, and the inside of a kitchen cupboard door (one that's opened frequently!) are good places to keep your list.

Also consider drafting a grocery list in the order in which the items are found in the store. Doing so can help you shop faster, because you won't find yourself running back and forth to pick up items you may have overlooked on the opposite side of the store. Doing a mental rundown of the aisles as you make your list also may prevent you from forgetting some of the things you need.

What to include on your weekly shopping list

The dairy-free foods listed here are those that are perishable and don't keep for more than a week or two. Photocopy the list and then pick and choose the foods you'd like to buy in any given week. Keep some extra copies of the list on hand just in case.

My suggestions for a weekly grocery list include the following:

- ❑ **Nondairy cheese**
    - ❑ Soy, rice, and nut milk varieties
    - ❑ Bricks and shredded varieties
    - ❑ Cheddar, Swiss, mozzarella, jack, and others
- ❑ **Nondairy coffee creamer (in pint and quart cartons)**
- ❑ **Nondairy cream cheese**
    - ❑ Plain
    - ❑ Flavored
- ❑ **Fresh deli items**
    - ❑ Veggie wrap sandwiches
    - ❑ Fresh pizza with veggie toppings (cheeseless)
    - ❑ Vinaigrette coleslaw (no milk-laced mayo)
- ❑ **Nondairy milk (in half-gallon cartons)**
    - ❑ Soy, rice, and almond
    - ❑ Plain (for cooking)
    - ❑ Flavored
- ❑ **Nondairy pudding cups**
- ❑ **Nondairy sour cream**
- ❑ **Soy yogurt**
    - ❑ Plain (as a sour cream substitute)
    - ❑ Fruited and flavored

What to include on your monthly shopping list

The following items keep for months in the cupboard, refrigerator, or freezer. You can buy them less often, and you can stock up when there's a sale.

❑ **Nondairy chocolate**

❑ **Nondairy frozen novelties**

  ❑ Frozen fruit bars

  ❑ Italian ice

  ❑ Nondairy ice cream bars

❑ **Nondairy ice cream**

  ❑ Soy, rice, and coconut milk varieties

  ❑ Nondairy sorbet

❑ **Nondairy margarine (trans-fat-free)**

❑ **Nondairy milk (in aseptic cartons)**

  ❑ Soy, rice, almond, and grain-based

  ❑ Plain (for cooking)

  ❑ Flavored

Knowing Where to Get What You Need

Many people have favorite stores where they go to buy specific items. For example, I prefer to go to my neighborhood co-op for the brand of nondairy margarine I like best (Earth Balance). Because supermarkets often don't carry it, I pick it up at the co-op when my supply is low and I happen to be there for something else.

Where you shop depends on your food preferences and the variety of stores in your area. In this section, I describe some of the most common types of stores that are likely to carry nondairy products you may want to use. I also provide some suggestions for getting those groceries you need if you don't see them at your local stores.

Your access to natural foods stores and co-ops that carry a wide variety of nondairy products may depend, in part, on where you live. People who live in larger cities, affluent communities, or college towns typically have the most options. People who live in small, rural communities usually have fewer choices, though they do have access to online stores.

Your local supermarket

The most obvious location you can shop for your food (nondairy included) is at your local supermarket. The good news about your neighborhood supermarket is that it has probably undergone a makeover in the past few years because of the transformation in the way people eat.

As a result of this makeover, you likely can find more and more healthy foods up and down the aisles. In fact, if you live in a big city, it's possible that your neighborhood supermarket carries a wide enough variety of nondairy products that you can do all or most of your shopping in one stop.

The natural foods industry — including organic foods — has seen a tremendous growth in popularity since the mid-1990s. The growth of that industry is what first brought more nondairy specialty products into mainstream supermarkets.

The soymilk, nondairy cheese, and other specialty foods that once were sold only in health food stores have moved into ordinary supermarkets. What's more, large multinational food companies have bought many of the small companies that once produced those foods. Those products now sit side by side with mainstream brands on the shelves in your local supermarket. All of this is good news for anyone interested in rice milk, almond milk, dairy-free coffee creamer, and soy yogurt.

Natural foods stores

If you've never before set foot in a natural foods store, it's time to do so. For anyone eating a dairy-free diet, natural foods stores are the guaranteed, one-stop shopping destination for all the nondairy foods and beverages you need. Most natural foods stores carry every item listed in the shopping lists included in this chapter. They also are a great place to go to sample a variety of different kinds of products and to compare brands.

Making friends with the store manager

If you're shopping for items on your grocery list and you don't see what you want, you have a friend who can help. In most stores, the store manager often is willing to place a special order if the store doesn't stock an item you want. All you have to do is ask. Depending on the product, you may even be able to get a discount if you order by the case. If you don't need that much of the item, get some friends to go in on with you.

Examples of large national chains include Whole Foods and Earth Fare in the Southeast. Local mom-and-pop natural foods stores also are still around, and Trader Joe's carries a fair number of nondairy specialty products such as soymilk, rice milk, and soy yogurt.

Other options

If your supermarket doesn't supply you with everything you need and you don't have a natural foods store close by, you also can find nondairy foods in a variety of other places. Here's a rundown of some of the choices you may have:

- ✔ **Warehouse stores:** Costco and Sam's Club are in the dairy-free game now. They carry at least a few nondairy specialty foods. Look for Silk soymilk as well as private-label brands.

- ✔ **Food cooperatives:** A *co-op* is an organization that buys foods in volume for its members. Because the group buys in volume, it often can pass along cost savings to co-op members. They usually stock products similar to those you find at natural foods stores. Many college towns have food co-ops.

- ✔ **Online sources:** For people who live in rural communities and other places where shopping options are limited, Web sites that sell specialty foods, including many nondairy products, can be a lifesaver. Two sources that cater to vegetarians and *vegans* (strict vegetarians who never eat dairy or other animal products) are the Mail Order Catalog for Healthy Eating (www.healthy-eating.com) and Food Fight (store.foodfightgrocery.com/index.html).

- ✔ **Specialty stores:** Gourmet stores and other upscale, specialty stores may surprise you from time to time with interesting nondairy products and products often found in natural foods stores.

- ✔ **Ethnic markets:** Asian, Indian, Middle Eastern, and other ethnic markets often carry foods such as condiments, frozen entrees, and packaged foods not commonly found in ordinary supermarkets.

Watching Your Budget While Taking Care of Your Health

Specialty products such as nondairy cheese and soy yogurt can be expensive to buy on a regular basis — especially the organic varieties (see the later section "Natural or Organic? Determining What's Best" for more information). To go dairy-free for the long run, you'd be wise to think of ways to economize.

The good news is that doing so isn't difficult. In this section, I share some ideas for controlling costs while enjoying your dairy-free diet and taking care of your body.

Making sure you have low-cost staples on hand

Although you may be accustomed to eating soy yogurt and drinking almond milk, plenty of other nondairy foods are available to round out your diet, and they don't have to cost a small fortune. Economize where you can so you can spend a little extra on specialty items like nondairy cream cheese and soy ice cream. You can economize by making some of these low-cost staples the foundations of more of your meals:

- **Canned beans:** Main dishes made with beans include black-eyed peas with rice, Cuban black beans, Creole-style beans, bean chili, bean burritos, bean nachos, and baked beans on whole-wheat toast.

- **Miscellaneous:** Hot and cold cereals, frozen and canned vegetables, and fresh, in-season produce are other healthful, good-value foods that can play a bigger role in more of your meals.

- **Pasta:** Whole-wheat varieties are the healthiest because they're high in fiber and nutrients.

- **Rice:** Pair rice with bean dishes or use it as the base for stir-fry and *paella,* a traditional Spanish-style dish made with steamed rice and vegetables. (Check out Chapter 11 for a recipe for Spanish Paella with Shrimp.)

- **Soup:** Make your own soup or buy canned (low sodium, when possible). Pair soup with whole-grain bread or a salad to make it a meal. Do be sure to check labels when buying soups, however. Some, especially the creamy varieties, can harbor hidden dairy ingredients.

Comparing prices

When you're shopping on a budget, one of the best ways to save a little money is to be a comparison shopper. In particular, compare the prices of name-brand, store-brand, and private-label products. Private-label and store-brand foods often cost substantially less than similar name-brand products. The quality often is just as good, too. Look for private-label and store-brand versions of soymilk, rice milk, soy yogurt, and other nondairy products. Compare prices of similar products between stores, too.

Check the unit pricing shown on the grocery shelves near each product. For example, unit pricing may show you the price per ounce of one product compared with another. Comparing unit prices can help you find the best values.

Considering versatile products

One way to be practical when buying nondairy specialty foods is to purchase varieties that can be used for more than one purpose. For example, soymilk and other forms of nondairy milk are typically sold in plain and flavored varieties. The flavored products, such as vanilla and chocolate flavors, usually are slightly sweetened. Although these sweetened varieties are tasty for drinking, they aren't always useful for cooking savory dishes.

For instance, when I make mashed potatoes, I usually add some milk and margarine to make the potatoes creamier. Adding vanilla-flavored almond milk to my potatoes just doesn't sound very appealing. Plain almond milk would be a better choice. Plus plain almond milk tastes pretty good on my breakfast cereal and in my coffee. By buying only one variety, I can open one container and use it for several purposes. Having two open containers increases the likelihood that one may spoil before I can use it all.

Nondairy cheese is another example. You're more likely to find multiple uses for cheddar- or mozzarella-style cheese than for pepper jack cheese.

Plan your week's menus to maximize your use of nondairy products with limited shelf lives. For example, if you buy a large container of plain soy yogurt, use part of it in baking or making a dip, and then use the remainder throughout the week with your breakfast or with fresh berries or baked potatoes.

Shopping for value

When shopping, you want to make sure you're spending your money wisely and not foolishly throwing it away. Here are a few ways you can save:

- ✔ **Buy in bulk.** When you purchase items in bulk, the prices usually are lower. Of course, it's not worth buying three half gallons of soymilk if they spoil before you can use them. If you can use larger quantities of certain items within a reasonable amount of time, though, buying in volume — in multipacks or case lots — can save you money at warehouse stores, supermarkets, and natural foods stores.

- ✔ **Use coupons.** The savings from coupons can add up depending on how many you use. Natural foods stores, co-ops, supermarkets, and warehouse stores often post coupons alongside products being promoted.

Or you can look at in-store circulars, mailers, and inside magazines sold at natural foods stores. However, don't purchase items just because you find a coupon for it.

✔ **Buy only what you'll use.** A block of soy cheese may cost less per ounce than cheese that already has been grated. However, if grating the cheese is a big barrier to your using it, then your expensive chunk of soy cheese may spoil and go to waste. The moral of this story? Spend the extra money to spring for the products you'll use.

Natural or Organic? Determining What's Best

Nondairy products such as soymilk, rice milk, and nondairy cheese have been regular features in natural foods stores for decades. Because the original market for these foods was rooted in the natural products industry, these foods tend to be labeled as being *natural* and also *organic*. You may be wondering exactly what these terms mean and whether they're important for people who want to live dairy-free. Don't worry. The following sections spell out these terms in plain English so you can understand them better.

Natural foods

Unfortunately, no legal definition for the term *natural foods* exists. However, within the natural foods industry, the general understanding is that natural foods are those that are as close to their natural state as possible. That means natural foods are minimally processed, and they contain no artificial colorings, flavorings, synthetic preservatives, and other substances that don't naturally occur in foods.

In general, you do well by buying natural foods. They tend to contain fewer of the substances that many people eat in excess (sodium, artificial ingredients, refined flour, artery-clogging trans fats, and others). They also tend to contain more dietary fiber and fewer added sweeteners.

Natural foods aren't always more nutritious, though. Natural candies, cakes, snack chips, and other treats can be just as devoid of nutrition as nonnatural junk foods. Natural nondairy frozen novelties such as ice cream bars and similar desserts contain few nutrients in exchange for the calories. Limit these foods and don't let them push more nutritious foods from your diet.

Organic foods

Organic is a term that for decades was self-defined — and self-regulated — by the natural foods industry, which adhered to high standards for the foods it sold. After much debate (see the nearby sidebar "The war over labeling foods organic,") companies that grow and process foods can get their products certified as organic through third-party state and private agencies that are accredited by the U.S. Department of Agriculture. Here's what the label and its variations mean:

- ✔ **100 Percent Organic:** All ingredients in foods with this label must meet the organic standards.

- ✔ **USDA Organic:** Products that contain at least 95 percent organic ingredients can use this label. The remaining 5 percent of the ingredients must be approved for use in organic products. In other words, no sewage sludge is allowed!

- ✔ **Organic ingredients:** Products with at least 70 percent organic ingredients can highlight that fact on the ingredient lists on package labels.

So how important is it that your nondairy foods be organic? The practical reality is that most of the specialty products you may want to buy — soymilk, rice milk, almond milk, soy yogurt, nondairy cheeses, and similar products — are already going to be grown and produced according to organic standards. That's the good news. The bad news is that organic products generally are more expensive.

All else being equal, however, you're better off eating organic foods because, compared to *conventional foods* — foods not produced using organic standards — they expose you to fewer environmental contaminants that can potentially raise your risk for health problems.

Beyond nondairy specialty food products, you may want to learn more about foods you should look for in their organic forms. A helpful tool for identifying the 12 fruits and vegetables most likely to be contaminated with potentially harmful amounts of pesticides, herbicides, and other substances is available from the nonprofit Environmental Working Group (EWG). A pocket guide to the dirty dozen — and an iPhone application — are available online from EWG at `www.foodnews.org/index.php`.

The war over labeling foods organic

In the early 1990s, a food fight broke out when large, multinational food companies decided to get into the natural and organic foods business. By that time, the general public had developed a great interest in natural and organic foods, driving up sales so much that big food companies found it advantageous to get on board.

The problems occurred when the newcomers tried to loosen the high standards previously maintained for organic foods by the natural foods industry. For example, big food companies wanted to save on costs by permitting foods grown in soil fertilized with sewage sludge to nevertheless be labeled organic.

After years of controversy and public debate, the conflict resulted in the U.S. Congress passing in 1990 the Organic Foods Production Act. In 2002, the U.S. Department of Agriculture implemented a final rule that established a nationally recognized set of organic standards. These standards uphold the original high standards set forth by the natural foods industry.

Chapter 8

Cooking Tips and Techniques

In This Chapter

▶ Using nondairy ingredients successfully

▶ Choosing helpful appliances to make cooking easier

▶ Working with new and traditional recipes

*Y*ou want to eliminate dairy from your diet, right? Otherwise you probably wouldn't be reading this book. If so, it's time for a cooking lesson. I want to share some tips and techniques with you because using nondairy forms of milk, cheese, and other dairy substitutes can greatly increase the number of foods available to you for your diet. It's worth your time to figure out how to use these products. Of course, that means more cooking from scratch at home.

Cooking for yourself — rather than relying on packaged or ready-made products — gives you much more control over the ingredients in your foods. Simple substitutions in traditional, dairy-containing recipes often are all you need to transform a dairy-full dish into a dairy-free option you can enjoy.

You need to know about some of the quirks associated with nondairy ingredients and how they behave in recipes as well as tips for modifying your approach to preparing recipes when you replace dairy products with nondairy alternatives. So, in this chapter, I provide a few tricks you should know. I also describe some kitchen appliances you may find especially useful and offer suggestions for creating your own recipe stash that's customized to suit your tastes.

It may take more time and planning to cook your own meals, but it's worth it. You'll save money, have more variety in your diet, and eat more healthfully. Aim to become your own dairy-free chef.

Noting Special Considerations for Cooking Dairy-Free

For the most part, nondairy ingredients work the same way that dairy products do. They can be swapped — cup for cup — for the milk, cheese, and other common dairy ingredients in your favorite recipes. However, I'd be remiss not to tell you about the few exceptions.

In some cases, nondairy ingredients need special handling for optimal results. Not to worry, though. You don't need high-level cooking skills or special fancy doodads to get it right. All you need to know are a few of the idiosyncrasies so you aren't disappointed (and don't waste money) when something doesn't turn out the way you'd hoped. So that's what I devote this section to: Tricks of the trade for working with nondairy ingredients.

Keep in mind, too, that manufacturers also have lots of helpful information — including recipes — on their Web sites to help you use their nondairy products. I get you started in this section, but you can find plenty more assistance if you need it. Just search for a company with your favorite Web browser.

Working with nondairy milks

As far as nondairy products go, milk substitutes are the big success story. As a general rule, they're terrific products. Cooking with soymilk, rice milk, almond milk, and other milk substitutes (coconut milk, nut milk, oat milk, hemp milk, potato milk, and so on) is a breeze. Making the substitution is simple: Use any nondairy milk cup for cup in place of cow's milk. The flavor, appearance, and texture of the foods you make will be the same.

Don't hesitate to use any of the nondairy substitutes in place of cow's milk for any baking and cooking needs, including in puddings, soups, and white sauces. They work very well. In most cases, you won't be able to tell the difference between foods made with nondairy milk instead of cow's milk.

When you use nondairy milk in cooking, you must keep a few points in mind. Milk substitutes are available in a range of flavors or as plain, unflavored varieties. The variety of milk you use depends on the type of recipe you're making. For example:

> ✔ **Use plain varieties for savory recipes.** If you use nondairy milk to make mashed potatoes, cream sauces, cream soups, scrambled eggs or omelets, and other foods that aren't sweet, don't use sweet milk — such as vanilla, chocolate, or other varieties that are slightly sweetened. Instead, use plain, unsweetened varieties of soymilk, rice milk, and almond milk.

The recipes for Cream of Tomato Soup and Creamed Potatoes with Brown Gravy in Chapter 10 are good illustrations of this principle.

If you aren't sure whether a particular milk is sweet, check the ingredient label. Many brands of flavored nondairy milk are sweetened with small amounts of evaporated cane juice. Others, such as some brands of rice milk, don't contain added sweeteners. Nevertheless, if they have vanilla flavoring added to them, they may not taste right in savory dishes. So, in general, stick to plain nondairy milks when you make foods that aren't sweet.

✔ **Use vanilla varieties for sweet recipes.** Vanilla nondairy milk works well in cookies, cakes, quick breads, muffins, pancakes, waffles, puddings you make from scratch (it doesn't work as well in instant pudding), smoothies, and any other foods in which you wouldn't mind a mildly sweet, vanilla flavor. Check out the recipes for Easy French Toast in Chapter 9 and Grandma's Tapioca Pudding in Chapter 14 as examples.

Save chocolate, cocoa-, or carob-flavored milks for recipes in which you wouldn't mind a chocolately flavor, such as in pancakes, waffles, pudding, and some cookies and muffins. The recipe for Favorite Chocolate Pudding in Chapter 14 is an example where chocolate soymilk or rice milk works well.

✔ **Expect to use plain and vanilla nondairy milks for most recipes because they're the most versatile varieties.** If you only want to keep one variety of nondairy milk on hand, buy plain, because it works in both sweet and savory recipes. If you like to use vanilla soymilk or rice milk on your breakfast cereal, and you may use it often in baked goods and other sweet foods, you may want to keep vanilla-flavored products in your refrigerator, ready to use. Then you also can keep an aseptic carton of plain milk on hand in the pantry for times when you need it. (Head to Chapter 6 for more information on the shelf life of nondairy milk in aseptic cartons.)

If a recipe calls for buttermilk, you can handle that in a nondairy fashion, too. Make your own by adding 2 teaspoons of lemon juice or vinegar to 1 cup of any milk substitute. Mix it well and let it stand for a few minutes before using.

Nondairy milk is versatile, but don't try to store it in the freezer. Freezing doesn't hurt the nutritional value or safety of the product, but it causes a substantial — and negative — change in the consistency of the product.

Cooking with dairy-free cheese

Nondairy cheese is coming into its own. In fact, products on the market today are far better than those that were available 10 or 20 years ago.

Still, you'll find considerable variability among products. Flavor, texture, and melt quality vary by brand and variety. So to find the brands that work best for you, you need to experiment with several before settling on your favorites.

The high fat content of most varieties of dairy cheese contributes significantly to their flavor and texture as well as to how easily they melt. Nondairy cheeses don't replicate those qualities. They do a good job, but you need to figure out how to choose the right nondairy cheese for your particular recipe.

Some general rules apply to using nondairy cheeses. For best results, keep this advice in mind:

- ✔ **Mix it up.** Nondairy cheese works best when it's used as one of several ingredients in a dish rather than as a stand-alone topper on a cracker. It works better when mixed with other ingredients because those other ingredients help compensate for the texture and lack of richness of most nondairy cheeses (as compared to full-fat dairy cheese). The Zucchini Parmesan in Chapter 11 illustrates this principle.

- ✔ **Help it melt.** When mixing nondairy cheese in with other ingredients in casseroles, soups, and pasta dishes, be sure to grate it. The other hot, moist ingredients in these foods help melt the cheese. Grated cheese has more surface area than it does in chunks or strips, so it melts more quickly and evenly than larger chunks of cheese. A good example of this tip in action is the Macaroni and Cheese recipe in Chapter 10.

- ✔ **Experiment.** Test soy-, rice- and nut-based varieties of nondairy cheese to see which you like best in various recipes. You may like the unique flavor, texture, or melting qualities of one variety over another.

Don't forget that you can make your own cheese, too. Mash a block of firm tofu and mix in a few teaspoons of lemon juice. Use this as a substitute for ricotta cheese or cottage cheese in recipes for lasagna and other pasta dishes, as well as in desserts such as Danish pastries and cheese blintzes. The recipes for Manicotti with Tofu, Spinach, and Mushrooms and Easy Vegetable Lasagna in Chapter 11 are two examples of how to use homemade cheese.

Incorporating dairy-free yogurt and sour cream

If you like to make your own dips, sauces, and desserts using yogurt and sour cream, you're in luck: The nondairy varieties of these foods work well as replacements for their dairy-based counterparts.

In general, nondairy varieties of yogurt and sour cream work best in recipes for cold foods, such as dips, spreads, dressings, and dessert fillings. In these recipes, the ingredients are simply blended or gently mixed with the other ingredients in the recipe. The Calypso Fruit Salad in Chapter 9 is one example. Nondairy yogurt and sour cream also work well in baked goods, such as cakes and quick breads. The recipe for Country Cornbread in Chapter 13 is an example.

The recipes to watch out for are those in which the nondairy yogurt or sour cream has a tendency to separate. A good example is when you make and heat sauces on the stovetop. Separation is a particular threat when you use nondairy yogurt.

If you do try your hand at making a cooked sauce, add the soy yogurt, sour cream, or other nondairy substitute gradually, stirring constantly. After the ingredient is blended well, don't overcook the sauce. If you cook it too long, the ingredients may break down and separate.

Naming the Appliances You Can Use

Although I resist the call for unnecessary appliances that take up precious kitchen counter space and collect to create an appliance graveyard in the pantry and kitchen cupboards (or maybe even in the basement), I do make use of several appliances that make my work faster and easier in the kitchen. In this section, I describe some appliances I think may be worth your money and space. These appliances are particularly useful for making many of the nondairy recipes I include in this book.

And while you're considering whether to invest in a few new appliances, take this opportunity to weed out any that are currently collecting dust. That bread machine or slow cooker may be a good starting point. If you haven't used them in several years, out they go. Donate them to a local charity or recycle them.

High-speed blenders

A high-speed blender is one of the most versatile appliances you can have in your dairy-free kitchen. If you're in the market for a blender, look for a high-quality model with a glass blender jar and heavy-duty blade. A blender (see Figure 8-1) mixes or purées food and comes in all sizes and shapes.

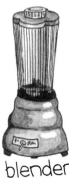

Figure 8-1:
A blender can help you in your dairy-free kitchen.

blender

High-speed blenders are great for a wide variety of tasks. You can use them to make everything from smoothies to soups. For example, I like to use my high-speed blender to whip up fresh fruit smoothies like the Very Cranberry Smoothie and Strawberry Kiwi Smoothie recipes in Chapter 14. To give homemade soups a creamy consistency, you can place a portion of the vegetables (and some liquid) from a batch of soup into the blender, purée, and then stir the puréed soup back into the pot (check out Chapter 10 for some soup recipes).

An advantage of a high-speed blender over a juicer — another popular appliance — is that it conserves the health-supporting dietary fiber in fruits and vegetables. Rather than separating the fiber from the juice, as most juicers do, blenders incorporate the pulp into the drink. Blenders also are easier to clean than most juicers. Juicers often have more parts to disassemble and more nooks and crannies that collect food and need cleaning.

On the downside, although ordinary high-speed kitchen blenders are relatively inexpensive, their motors tend to overheat easily when the blender is used to process thick mixtures. The recipe for Spinach and Artichoke Hummus in Chapter 12, for example, can be a challenge for an ordinary kitchen blender.

Instead, a heavy-duty, restaurant-quality blender, such as the Vita-Mix, holds an advantage over ordinary blenders because it has a larger capacity and more powerful motor. My own Vita-Mix is more than 15 years old and going strong, on its original motor, and is a reliable tool for making thick dips and sauces as well as smoothies and soup. The trade-off is that the Vita-Mix is much more expensive than ordinary kitchen blenders. Take that into consideration as you weigh the practicality of buying one. If you use it often, though, you'll be glad to have the higher-quality appliance.

If you need any more convincing, here's one example of the many simple dairy-free foods you can whip up in minutes with a heavy-duty blender: In the summertime, make cold melon soup by placing fresh cantaloupe or honeydew chunks, plain soy yogurt, and a few teaspoons of honey in a blender and blend until creamy. For thinner soup, add orange or apple juice by the tablespoon until the soup reaches your desired consistency. Pour it into a rimmed soup bowl and serve it with a dash of cinnamon or nutmeg and a sprig of fresh mint on top.

Food processors: Large and small

If you spend much time at all in the kitchen, you'll appreciate owning a food processor. A food processor is similar to a blender in that it can cut up foods quickly and mix dough and other ingredients with ease. The bowls on most food processors, though, aren't meant to process large amounts of liquid, whereas blenders include jars with pour spouts. Unlike blenders, food processors can thinly slice fruits and vegetables and grate cheese or carrots. Blenders are better at chopping or making purées. So the functions of food processors and blenders are different. For a fully stocked kitchen, you need both appliances.

A food processor can make you look like a professional chef with its precision-slicing ability. It also can cut down substantially on the time and muscle it takes to prep ingredients — it can chop and slice foods in a fraction of the time it would take you to do it by hand.

Foodies like to keep two types of food processors (see Figure 8-2) on hand:

✔ **A large, full-sized food processor for heavy-duty jobs:** Full-sized food processors not only make quick work of larger chopping jobs, but they also yield results that are more consistent than when chopping is done by hand. Larger, full-sized food processors are incredibly helpful for preparing amounts of ingredients for casseroles, salads, and other dishes. You can find a full-sized food processor helpful, for example, in preparing the Confetti Cole Slaw in Chapter 10 or the Spinach and Basil Pesto Sauce in Chapter 12.

✔ **A small-capacity version for small jobs:** Small-capacity food processors, or *mini food processors,* have a 1- or 2-cup capacity. They can be helpful in grating, mincing, and chopping small amounts quickly. You can use one for processing tiny amounts of herbs, nuts, or other minor ingredients in recipes (why dirty the big machine when the little one will do?). For example, I use mine to grate carrots and a small chunk of red cabbage for color in a salad, to grate small amounts of nondairy cheese, or to chop onions if I don't want to do it by hand.

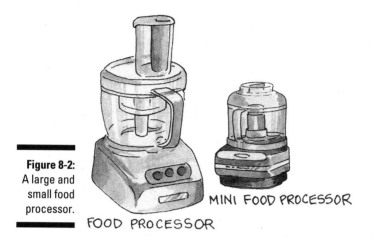

Figure 8-2:
A large and small food processor.

MINI FOOD PROCESSOR

FOOD PROCESSOR

The food processor is the perfect kitchen tool to use for making fresh *gazpacho* — a cold, traditional Spanish soup made with fresh summer vegetables from your garden. You can make many variations of this dish, but most of them include one or more of the following fresh, uncooked ingredients, blended until smooth: tomatoes, onions, cucumbers, bell peppers, celery, olive oil, chives, minced garlic, red wine vinegar, and lemon juice. Not a drop of dairy. A quick Web search can turn up lots of gazpacho variations to try.

Mixers

Sometimes mixing something by hand just isn't enough. In this case, you need an electric mixer. Mixers come in the following two primary varieties (see Figure 8-3):

✔ **Small, hand-held mixers:** Hand mixers are convenient and easy to use. They're also small enough to be stored in a kitchen drawer. They work well when you have a small job to do quickly, such as whipping creamed potatoes with a little bit of margarine and plain soymilk or mixing a small batch of cookie dough or cake batter. Small, hand-held mixers are inexpensive and nice to have on hand.

Be sure to match the job to the right appliance. Thick doughs and other mixing jobs that require a lot of power may be too much for the motors on many hand-held mixers and may cause them to burn out. For heavy-duty jobs, use an upright, full-sized mixer.

✔ **Full-sized, counter-top mixers:** Your grandmother may have called her full-size mixer her "Mixmaster." My heavy-duty Kitchen Aid mixer also is an example. While full-sized food processors can serve many of the same purposes as full-sized mixers, you may find the mixer more convenient to use when you're making cookies and cakes.

Counter-top mixers do a good job of creaming cookie and cake batters, and they're simpler to take apart and clean than food processors. On the other hand, you can't use a mixer to chop vegetables or process garbanzo beans.

A heavy-duty mixer shares many of the same uses as a full-sized food processor. So if you have either, you may not need the other. On the other hand, the two appliances also have some differences in their applicability to certain tasks. For that reason, I recommend keeping both. When it comes down to it, your choice of counter-top mixer versus full-sized food processor is a matter of personal preference. Take your choice, or take both.

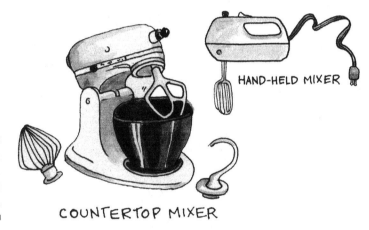

HAND-HELD MIXER

Figure 8-3:
A small and full-sized mixer.

COUNTERTOP MIXER

Ice cream machines

Electric ice cream machines (see Figure 8-4) are fun kitchen appliances to have. They're a good way to save money if you like to eat frozen desserts. Nondairy ice cream products are widely available in natural foods stores and many supermarkets, but they can be expensive. So why not make your own and save some money? Good-quality electric ice cream machines are available for as little as $40. Use them to make dairy-free fruit sorbet, sherbet, and ice cream.

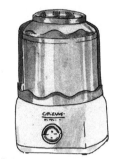

Figure 8-4:
An electric ice cream maker can make your favorite frozen desserts.

ELECTRIC ICE CREAM MAKER

Making your own frozen desserts can be especially helpful when you or one of your family members has a preference for soymilk, rice milk, almond milk, or any of the other nondairy forms of milk available. You can make the ice cream with your milk substitute of choice or use up odd bits of whatever may be languishing in your refrigerator.

Be creative and experiment with different flavors and additions, such as carob chips, mint flavoring, berries, coconut, chopped nuts, and others. I include several recipes in Chapter 14 for dairy-free ice cream, including strawberry or chocolate, which are made with tofu. I also include a recipe for a version made with rice milk, though you can substitute any variety of nondairy milk you prefer.

Recipe Magic: Adapting Your Favorites

You may have a difficult time imagining a milkshake without ice cream or a cream soup without whole milk. Or maybe you've never tried nachos made with melted cheddar-style rice cheese. The dairy ingredients you've traditionally used — over and over again — to cook and bake with perform certain functions in recipes. Cheese adds bulk and binds ingredients together. Milk can make foods brown and also adds moisture. So it may come as a surprise to you to realize how many of these functions can be duplicated with other nondairy ingredients.

For instance, I think about the time I spent on a tiny island near Fiji, where I ate a breakfast dish covered with a thick, white cream sauce — made with coconut milk. Or the big bowl of hot, hearty cream of potato soup I once ate at a vegetarian restaurant in New York City. I was stunned to discover that tofu was the secret ingredient that gave this creamy, dairy-free soup its thick consistency.

In this section, I share some advice for branching out on your own and experimenting with using new ingredients to make old favorite foods — and some new ones, too.

Adjusting traditional recipes

Chances are good that when you swap nondairy ingredients for dairy-based ingredients in traditional recipes, you won't always notice a difference in the flavor, texture, or appearance of the food. That's especially true when you use nondairy milk in place of cow's milk.

However, sometimes you may still notice some subtle differences in foods when you alter recipes. Those differences depend on the ingredients used in the original recipe and how closely the qualities of substitute ingredients match the original.

For example, using almond milk or soymilk instead of cow's milk may give a smoothie or pudding a slightly different flavor than the same foods made with cow's milk. And using melted, rice-based, cheddar-style cheese substitute instead of full-fat dairy cheddar cheese on a plate of nachos may lend a different texture and appearance to the finished product. The rice cheese may not melt as completely as the dairy cheese, or it may have a slightly different consistency. Different isn't necessarily better or worse. It's just different. Different can be good.

As you begin living dairy-free, expect to experiment with recipes until you figure out which substitutions work for you and which ones don't. You'll encounter a few duds along the way, but you'll also discover some new favorites. Everyone has different food preferences, and what I like may not be the same as what you like.

Keeping notes as you cook

As you experiment with changes to your favorite traditional recipes and try new ones, take notes about what works and what doesn't. At the time, you may think you'll remember the changes, but chances are good that you may forget when you're making the recipe again later. Your notes also may be helpful to someone else who may try their hand at your recipe.

Jot notes to yourself in pencil in the margins of cookbook pages or on recipe cards. Note on the original recipe the substitutions you made and how much of each ingredient you used. Include observations about the look, smell, and consistency as you cook it.

When you finish a dish, jot down how it tastes and make notes about ideas for possible improvements or minor adjustments you may want to try next time. When you fix the recipe again and make an adjustment, erase and update your previous notes; think of your recipes as works in progress.

Creating your own recipes

You may enjoy experimenting with recipes enough to create a collection of your own to share with family and friends. Creating your own recipes and cooking your own meals is liberating; it's the ultimate way of customizing your diet to meet your needs and preferences. If you're confident and want to create some of your own, you can go one of two routes:

- ✔ **Start from scratch.** If you're a confident cook, you know which ingredients go well together, how flavors complement and blend with each other, how to use more or less of various ingredients, and how to apply basic cooking techniques to get the results you want. If this description fits your cooking style, you can develop your own concoctions, combining ingredients in a variety of ways to get pleasing results.

- ✔ **Build on other recipes.** You may go this route if you want a little help. Or perhaps you don't have the time to experiment. If so, get a head start and create your own recipes by building on others that have been tested.

  If you want to try this method, identify any recipe that you've tried and liked. Think about ways to add to the recipe, or ingredients that can be swapped for others. For example, you may like the recipe in Chapter 10 for Creamy Potato and Leek Soup. Consider that recipe as your base, and then make some additions of your own. Throw in a handful of cooked, grated carrots and chopped spinach for extra texture. Use your imagination and create your own signature set of dairy-free recipes.

Part III
Meals Made Easy: Recipes for Everyone

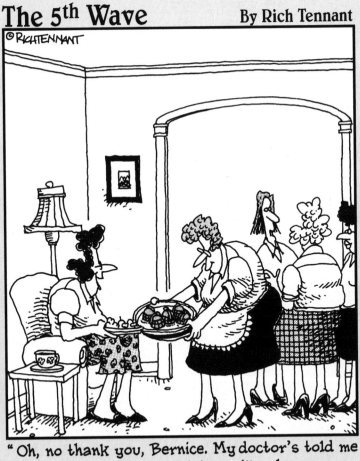

The 5th Wave   By Rich Tennant

"Oh, no thank you, Bernice. My doctor's told me to avoid foods containing milk, cheese, or hand grenades."

In this part . . .

Don't let your avoidance of dairy products stop you from creating delicious and healthful meals that your whole family will love. The recipes I include in this part are only a sample of the wide range of options available.

Fixing dairy-free foods can be simple and quick — notice the short ingredient lists and simple preparation instructions in my recipes. None of the recipes I include in this book require more than basic cooking skills.

I also aim for the recipes to be consistent with general advice for a health-supporting diet. The recipes I share are designed to help encourage more dietary fiber, fruits, vegetables, and whole grains, and less meat, sodium, saturated fat, trans fat, and added sugars.

Chapter 9

Waking Up to Breakfast Basics

In This Chapter

▶ Beginning with breakfast beverages

▶ Replacing milk and cheese in old breakfast standards

▶ Whipping up dairy-free, whole-grain favorites

*W*hether you like breakfast a little or a lot, taking time to eat in the morning is a smart way to start the day. Eating breakfast — even if it's nothing more than a glass of juice and a slice of toast — gives you an energy lift as you begin your day and helps you stay alert and perform your best all day long.

You may wonder, though, whether you can go dairy-free at breakfast. What can you eat to replace the milk in your cereal, the cream in your coffee, and the bowl of yogurt with granola? No problem. Making your breakfast dairy-free is easy. The same is true even when you have the time or inclination to fix a heartier breakfast spread. Most breakfast classics, including egg dishes and waffles and pancakes, can easily be made without dairy ingredients.

If you don't believe me, see for yourself. In this chapter, I include a variety of breakfast favorites to get you started.

Starting with Cold and Hot Beverages

Nothing is more energizing than starting the day off with a glass of cold, fresh fruit juice or a comforting mug of something creamy and warm. The recipes I share in this section are nice additions to the standard orange juice, coffee, and tea that, like these drinks, are already dairy-free.

Consider buying a juicer so you can make your own fresh fruit and vegetable juice mixtures at home. The options range from a simple vise for squeezing citrus fruits to more expensive machines that can liquefy carrots, spinach, celery, and other foods. Freshly squeezed juice is a dairy-free beverage alternative that's packed with vitamins and minerals. Fresh juice mixtures can be expensive to buy ready-made, so making your own at home not only ensures freshness but can save you money, too. If your juicer removes the pulp from the fruits and vegetables, conserve this healthful source of dietary fiber by adding it to soups or baked goods.

Masala Chai Tea

Masala chai — often called "chai" for short — is a delicious and fragrant traditional hot beverage from India made by brewing tea with spices, milk, and a sweetener. Recipes vary greatly among families. In this version, cow's milk is replaced with soymilk.

Preparation time: *15 minutes*

Yield: *Four 1-cup servings*

3 cups water

2 cinnamon sticks

6 cardamom pods

6 whole cloves

¼ inch of gingerroot, peeled and sliced thinly
(refer to Figure 9-1)

Several peppercorns

¼ cup loose black tea (such as Darjeeling)

1 cup plain or vanilla soymilk

3 tablespoons sugar

1 Combine the water, spices, and tea in a 2-quart saucepan. Cook over high heat until boiling. Turn off the heat and let the mixture steep for at least 10 minutes.

2 Strain the tea mixture and discard the spices. Add the soymilk and sugar to the strained tea mixture and stir well.

3 Reheat the tea until piping hot and serve.

Vary It! *Make your own signature variations by adding other spices, such as vanilla, almond, nutmeg, bay leaves, anise, or fennel and allspice. Check out Figure 9-2 for the many different spices used in this tea. Add extra soymilk if the tea brews too strongly for your taste.*

Per serving: *Calories 57 (11 from Fat); Fat 1g (Saturated 0g); Cholesterol 0mg; Sodium 7mg; Carbohydrate 11g (Dietary Fiber 1g); Protein 2g.*

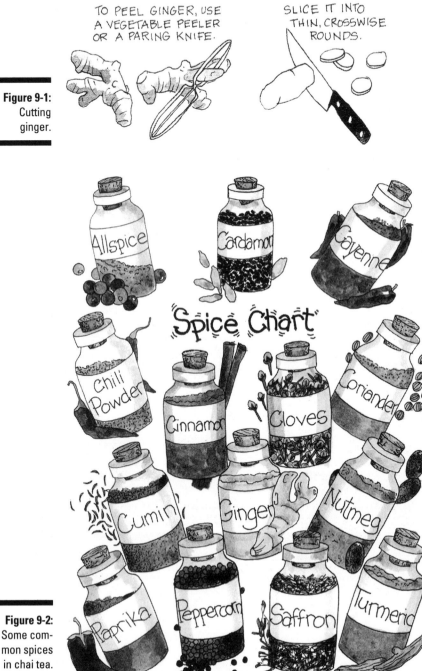

SLICING PEELED GINGER

TO PEEL GINGER, USE A VEGETABLE PEELER OR A PARING KNIFE.

SLICE IT INTO THIN, CROSSWISE ROUNDS.

Figure 9-1: Cutting ginger.

Spice Chart

Allspice

Cardamon

Cayenne

Chili Powder

Cinnamon

Cloves

Coriander

Cumin

Ginger

Nutmeg

Paprika

Peppercorn

Saffron

Turmeric

Figure 9-2: Some common spices in chai tea.

Juicy Jump-Start

Brightly hued carrot juice gives this mixture an added punch of color. That's why this juice looks so pretty when served in a glass pitcher or in stemmed glasses. Pineapple juice adds extra sweetness. A glass of this simple mixture is packed with vitamins C and A. Adjust the proportions of the juices to suit your taste.

Preparation time: *3 minutes*

Chilling time: *2 hours, or simply pour the beverage over ice*

Yield: *Four 1-cup servings*

*2 cups freshly squeezed orange juice
(2 to 3 medium oranges; see Figure 9-3
on how to juice an orange)*

1 cup fresh carrot juice

*1 cup of pineapple juice
(canned pineapple juice is okay)*

Several mint leaves

1 Combine juices in a glass pitcher and stir gently to mix thoroughly.

2 Chill for an hour or two before serving, if desired.

3 Pour into serving glasses and garnish each glass with mint leaves.

Vary It! *Replace all or part of the pineapple juice or carrot juice with orange juice or fresh spinach liquefied in a juicer. Play with the proportions to get the flavor as you like it.*

Per serving: *Calories 104 (4 from Fat); Fat 0g (Saturated 0g); Cholesterol 0mg; Sodium 33mg; Carbohydrate 25g (Dietary Fiber 1g); Protein 2g.*

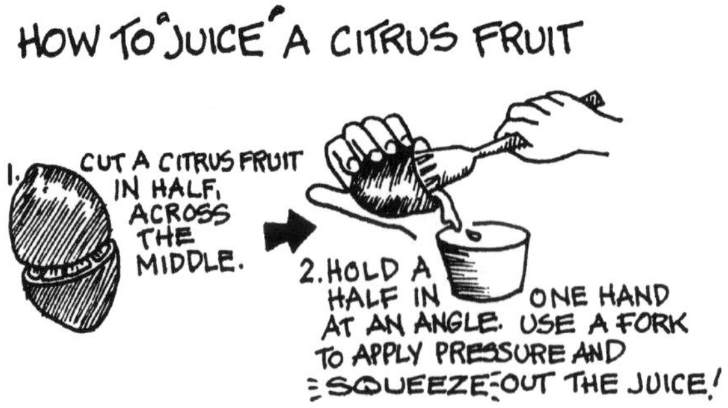

HOW TO "JUICE" A CITRUS FRUIT

Figure 9-3:
Use a fork to juice citrus fruit.

1. CUT A CITRUS FRUIT IN HALF, ACROSS THE MIDDLE.

2. HOLD A HALF IN ONE HAND AT AN ANGLE. USE A FORK TO APPLY PRESSURE AND SQUEEZE-OUT THE JUICE!

Montana Morning Mocha Joe

Coffee or cocoa? For cold-weather comfort, go for both. Adjust the proportions of coffee to cocoa to suit your tastes. This recipe calls for *unsweetened cocoa,* which is a fine powder made from cocoa solids that have been pressed out of chocolate liquor. Natural unsweetened cocoa powder is dark brown in color and gives a rich, chocolately flavor to hot chocolate drinks, brownies, and cakes. *Dutch-processed* cocoa powder is processed to neutralize the acidity of natural cocoa, and the result is a lighter-colored product with a mild chocolate flavor used in other recipes. Both of these forms of cocoa are naturally dairy-free. However, don't confuse them with hot cocoa mixes, which often contain added sugar and dairy ingredients.

Preparation time: *10 minutes*

Yield: *8 servings*

6 cups freshly brewed, strong coffee	*4½ cups plain or vanilla soymilk*
⅓ cup natural unsweetened cocoa powder	*½ teaspoon pure vanilla extract (optional if using vanilla soymilk)*
⅓ cup sugar	
1½ cups water	

1 Begin brewing the coffee.

2 Meanwhile, prepare the hot cocoa by combining the cocoa, sugar, and water in a 3-quart saucepan.

3 Heat until boiling, stirring frequently, and then boil for 2 minutes, stirring constantly.

4 Stir in the soymilk and continue to heat and stir until steaming hot.

5 Remove from the heat. Add the vanilla (if desired) and stir briskly with a whisk before serving.

6 Using a ladle, scoop ½ cup of the hot cocoa into a mug and then fill the mug the remainder of the way with coffee. Stir and serve.

Vary It! As an evening dessert beverage, add coconut-, caramel-, or Irish mint–flavored syrup.

Per serving: *Calories 90 (28 from Fat); Fat 3g (Saturated 1g); Cholesterol 0mg; Sodium 21mg; Carbohydrate 13g (Dietary Fiber 3g); Protein 5g.*

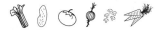

Leaving the Dairy Out of Classic Breakfast Dishes

Fixing a classic breakfast dish without using the common dairy ingredients that often are used in traditional recipes is so easy. Several of the recipes in this section are ideal for using soy and other forms of nondairy cheese because the cheese is distributed throughout the hot, moist egg mixture, helping it to melt evenly. Try the following recipes to whip up some of your breakfast favorites with dairy-free alternatives.

Spinach and Soy Cheese Quiche

This delicious dish can be served for breakfast or lunch, and the leftovers are good reheated. Use a whole-wheat pie shell, if possible, for the best flavor. If you serve this brunch favorite to a crowd, it will taste so good most folks won't even realize you've made it with dairy-free ingredients.

Preparation time: *25 minutes*

Cooking time: *35 minutes*

Yield: *6 servings*

3 tablespoons olive oil

1 medium onion, chopped (refer to Figure 9-4 for instruction)

10 ounces frozen, chopped spinach, thawed and thoroughly drained (or use 6 cups fresh spinach, chopped)

½ teaspoon salt

1 teaspoon lemon juice

4 eggs (or equivalent amount of cholesterol-free egg replacer)

1 cup plain soymilk

6 ounces nondairy Swiss-style cheese, grated

½ teaspoon black pepper

½ teaspoon ground nutmeg

One 9-inch pie shell (not deep-dish), unbaked (If using a ready-made shell, read the label. Some may contain skim milk solids or other dairy byproducts.)

Paprika

Tomato slices and flat-leaf parsley for garnish (optional)

1 Preheat the oven to 350 degrees.

2 In a medium skillet, heat the olive oil. Add the onions and cook over medium heat for about 2 minutes, or until onions become soft and translucent.

3 Add the spinach, salt, and lemon juice. Stir, cover the skillet, and cook the mixture over medium heat for 10 minutes. Take care not to burn the spinach. Remove from the heat and set aside.

4 Break the eggs into a medium bowl and beat them lightly with a fork or whisk. Add the soymilk, cheese, black pepper, and nutmeg, and then add the spinach mixture. Stir to combine.

5 Pour the filling mixture into the pie shell (which is in a pie pan). Top with a few shakes of paprika for color.

6 Place the quiche in the preheated oven and bake for 35 minutes, or until browned on top. Test for doneness by inserting a toothpick or knife in the center. When it comes out clean, the quiche is done.

7 Remove the quiche from the oven and let it stand for 10 minutes. Garnish with tomato slices and parsley sprigs, if desired, and serve hot.

Vary It! *If you don't have Swiss-style cheese on hand, feel free to substitute another variety of nondairy cheese, and omit the nutmeg. Add other ingredients — sundried tomatoes, sautéed mushrooms, soy-based bacon, or chopped black olives — in Step 4 as desired.*

Per serving: *Calories 349 (209 from Fat); Fat 23g (Saturated 6g); Cholesterol 148mg; Sodium 408mg; Carbohydrate 23g (Dietary Fiber 2g); Protein 14g.*

How to Chop an Onion

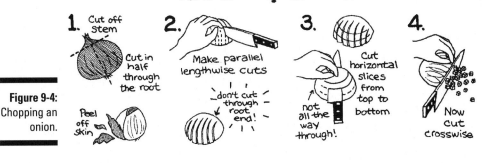

Figure 9-4: Chopping an onion.

Calypso Fruit Salad

Fruit salad is a quick, light breakfast by itself, or you can make it heartier by scooping it into a bowl of hot or cold cereal. As a side dish with pancakes, waffles, and egg dishes, it becomes an attractive accompaniment.

Preparation time: *10 minutes*

Chilling time: *2 hours*

Yield: *6 servings*

2 cups cubed watermelon

2 cups peeled, diced mango (refer to Figure 9-5)

1 cup pineapple chunks (drained, if using canned pineapple)

2 medium peeled and sliced bananas

¼ cup unsweetened coconut flakes

Several fresh mint leaves, chopped

6 ounces vanilla- or lemon-flavored soy yogurt

1 Place prepared fruits, coconut, and fresh mint in a medium-sized bowl and mix gently using a wooden spoon.

2 Chill mixture for at least 2 hours.

3 Add a dollop of yogurt on top of each dish of fruit salad upon serving.

Vary It! *Substitute other seasonal fruits as desired. Amounts don't have to be precise.*

Per serving: *Calories 149 (29 from Fat); Fat 3g (Saturated 2g); Cholesterol 0mg; Sodium 7 mg; Carbohydrate 31g (Dietary Fiber 4g); Protein 2g.*

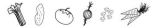

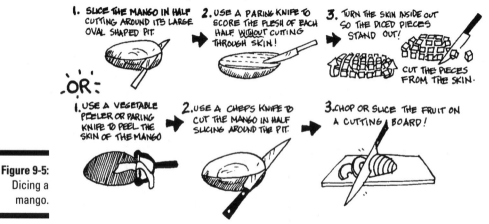

TWO WAYS TO CUT A MANGO...

1. SLICE THE MANGO IN HALF CUTTING AROUND ITS LARGE OVAL SHAPED PIT.

2. USE A PARING KNIFE TO SCORE THE FLESH OF EACH HALF WITHOUT CUTTING THROUGH SKIN!

3. TURN THE SKIN INSIDE OUT SO THE DICED PIECES STAND OUT!

CUT THE PIECES FROM THE SKIN.

:OR:

1. USE A VEGETABLE PEELER OR PARING KNIFE TO PEEL THE SKIN OF THE MANGO

2. USE A CHEF'S KNIFE TO CUT THE MANGO IN HALF SLICING AROUND THE PIT.

3. CHOP OR SLICE THE FRUIT ON A CUTTING BOARD!

Figure 9-5:
Dicing a mango.

Soy Cheese and Mushroom Scramble (with Soy-Based Bacon or Sausage)

This cheesy egg dish is versatile. It's delicious served over toasted sourdough bread. You also can heat leftovers in the microwave and use them as filling for on-the-go, whole-wheat pita pocket breakfast sandwiches.

Preparation time: *Less than 5 minutes; more if you have to grate the cheese*

Cooking time: *5 to 10 minutes*

Yield: *3 servings*

6 eggs (or equivalent amount of cheeseless, cholesterol-free egg replacer)

¼ cup plain soymilk

2 tablespoons olive oil

1 cup sliced, canned mushrooms, drained

¼ cup soy-based bacon, crumbled, or ⅓ cup soy sausage, crumbled (optional)

6 ounces cheddar-style soy cheese, grated (Caution: Read the label; some brands contain casein.)

Tomato slices and flat-leaf parsley for garnish (optional)

1 Break the eggs into a medium bowl and beat them lightly with a fork or whisk. Stir in the milk to combine.

2 In a medium skillet, heat ½ tablespoon of the olive oil. Add the mushrooms and cook for 2 to 3 minutes, until tender and some liquid has been released. Don't brown the mushrooms. Remove them from the pan. Add the remaining tablespoon and a half of oil to the same pan. Heat and then add the egg mixture and cook over low to medium heat for about 1 minute, until the bottom of the egg mixture is set and the top is still creamy-soft. Sprinkle the mushrooms and soy meat (if desired) into the egg mixture.

3 Using a flexible spatula, gently run the spatula all around the edges of the egg mixture to loosen it. Cut the egg mixture into thirds, and moving around the skillet, lift sections of the egg mixture with the spatula, turning them over as you go. After you've turned all the egg mixture, sprinkle the cheese over the top of it and cook for another minute until the eggs are completely set.

4 Transfer the eggs to a bowl or individual serving plates. Garnish with tomato slices and parsley (if desired) and serve immediately.

Vary It! *Experiment with different fillings. You can replace mushrooms and cheese with equal amounts of diced, cooked vegetables, such as onions, green peppers, roasted red peppers, artichoke hearts, black olives, or sundried tomatoes. You also can experiment with different types of nondairy cheese, such as pepper jack, mozzarella-style, and Swiss-style.*

Per serving: *Calories 366 (230 from Fat); Fat 26g (Saturated 4g); Cholesterol 425mg; Sodium 957mg; Carbohydrate 4g (Dietary Fiber 1g); Protein 28g. With the sausage: Calories 414 (261 From Fat); Fat 29g (Saturated 5g); Cholesterol 425mg; Sodium 1,125mg; Carbohydrate 5g (Dietary Fiber 2g); Protein 31g.*

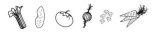

Working with Waffles, Pancakes, and Other Grains

You may have thought that dairy-free waffles, pancakes, French toast, and oatmeal weren't possible. The good news is they are. They taste the same as their lactose-laden cousins. Just use your favorite traditional recipes and substitute your choice of nondairy milk for the cow's milk. Or, if you're on the hunt for some new sweet breakfast recipes check out the ones I provide in this section.

Cranberry Walnut Oatmeal

This cereal is one of the healthiest ways you can jump-start a new day. The combination of nuts, dried berries, spices, and oatmeal is satisfying and delicious.

Preparation time: *5 minutes*

Cooking time: *5 minutes*

Yield: *Two 1-cup servings*

¾ cup water

1 cup quick-cooking rolled oats

¼ cup dried cranberries

¼ cup chopped walnuts

1 teaspoon cinnamon

1 cup vanilla soymilk (or your choice of nondairy milk, plain or vanilla)

2 tablespoons brown sugar

Additional soymilk as desired

1 Bring the water to a boil in a medium-sized saucepan.

2 Add the oats and boil for 1 minute, stirring constantly.

3 Add the cranberries, walnuts, cinnamon, soymilk, and brown sugar and cook on low heat for an additional 2 to 3 minutes, or until heated through. The mixture will be thick and creamy.

4 Remove from the heat and ladle into serving bowls. Serve with additional soymilk and extra cinnamon or brown sugar as desired.

Vary It! *Dice a peeled Granny Smith apple and add the apples with the water in Step 1. Then add the oats and the remaining ingredients and cook as directed.*

Per serving: Calories 420 (127 from Fat); Fat 14g (Saturated 2g); Cholesterol 0mg; Sodium 52mg; Carbohydrate 67g (Dietary Fiber 6g); Protein 11g.

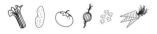

Multigrain Waffles

These dairy-free waffles are easy to make. They're light and fluffy and have a mild, nutty flavor. Follow the cooking instructions on your waffle iron for best results.

Preparation time: *10 minutes*

Cooking time: *40 minutes*

Yield: *5 Belgian-style waffles*

Special equipment: *Belgian waffle iron*

⅔ cup whole-wheat flour

⅔ cup all-purpose flour

½ cup rolled oats, quick cooking or regular

¼ cup wheat germ or corn meal

¼ cup packed brown sugar

1½ teaspoons baking soda

½ teaspoon baking powder

¼ teaspoon salt

2 teaspoons ground cinnamon

2 cups soymilk (or your choice of nondairy milk, plain or vanilla)

2 tablespoons vegetable oil

2 large eggs, slightly beaten (or equivalent amount of cholesterol-free egg replacer)

2 teaspoons pure vanilla extract

½ cup chopped pecans (optional)

Nonstick vegetable oil spray

1 Preheat the waffle iron and spray with vegetable oil. Meanwhile, measure the dry ingredients into a medium-sized bowl. Stir to combine.

2 Add the soymilk, oil, eggs, and vanilla and stir well using a whisk. The batter may be a bit lumpy, so don't overmix. Doing so may make the waffles tough. Stir in the chopped pecans, if desired.

3 Pour the batter by ¾-cup measures onto the hot, oiled waffle iron. (Spray the waffle iron with additional nonstick vegetable oil spray between each waffle to prevent sticking.) The batter should cover about three-fourths of the surface of a standard 8-inch square waffle iron. Cook until waffles are crispy and golden brown, about 5 minutes each. Repeat until all the batter is used. As you make the waffles, place the cooked ones on a warm plate until ready to serve.

Tip: *Leftover waffles can be refrigerated for two or three days and reheated in a toaster. Leftovers also can be sealed in an airtight container and frozen for several weeks before reheating.*

Per serving: *Calories 324 (99 from Fat); Fat 11g (Saturated 2g); Cholesterol 85mg; Sodium 575mg; Carbohydrate 46g (Dietary Fiber 6g); Protein 12g.*

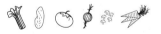

Blueberry Pecan Pancakes

The beaten egg whites provide the lift that makes these pancakes light, yet hearty. Leftover pancakes keep well in the refrigerator or freezer and can be reheated in the microwave oven.

Preparation time: *10 minutes*

Cooking time: *5 minutes*

Yield: *8 pancakes, or 4 servings*

1 cup whole-wheat flour

½ cup white flour

⅓ cup wheat germ or corn meal

1 teaspoon baking soda

1 teaspoon cinnamon

1 tablespoon baking powder

½ teaspoon salt

1¾ cups soymilk (or your choice of nondairy milk, plain or vanilla)

¼ cup vegetable oil

1 whole egg (or equivalent amount of cholesterol-free egg replacer)

¾ cup fresh blueberries

¼ cup chopped pecans

2 egg whites (or equivalent amount of cholesterol-free egg replacer), beaten stiff

Nonstick vegetable oil spray

1 Measure the dry ingredients into a medium-sized bowl.

2 Add the soymilk, oil, and whole egg, and stir well using a whisk. Break up any remaining chunks of flour by using the back of a spoon.

3 Fold in the blueberries and pecans with a wooden spoon or rubber spatula. Fold in the beaten egg whites. The batter will be thick but light and somewhat foamy.

4 Coat a griddle or 12-inch skillet with nonstick vegetable oil spray and preheat.

5 Pour the batter by ⅓-cup measures onto the hot, oiled griddle. When the pancakes are bubbly all over and the edges are browned, turn them over and cook on the remaining sides for about 30 seconds, or until the undersides are browned. Serve immediately.

Tip: *Egg whites are beaten stiff when they have thickened enough to form a peak when you pull the beaters out of the bowl. If you keep beating egg whites past this point, they can collapse and become thin again. The key is to stop beating when you notice that the whites are forming soft peaks that can stand up on their own.*

Remember: *Make the pancakes as soon as possible after mixing the batter, because the leavening action of the baking powder begins as soon as it mixes with the liquid ingredients. Batter left too long begins to lose its leavening power and can result in flat, dense pancakes.*

Per serving: Calories 444 (219 from Fat); Fat 24g (Saturated 2g); Cholesterol 53mg; Sodium 950mg; Carbohydrate 46g (Dietary Fiber 8g); Protein 16g.

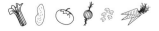

Easy French Toast

Use your imagination and experiment with different kinds of bread when you make this recipe. The basic recipe calls for whole-wheat bread, but it also works well using cinnamon, sourdough, multigrain, French, pumpkin, and banana breads, too. You also can experiment with different types and flavors of nondairy milk. Vanilla-flavored almond milk or soymilk is especially good in this recipe.

Preparation time: *10 minutes*

Cooking time: *About 6 minutes*

Yield: *Three 2-slice servings*

2 eggs (or equivalent amount of cholesterol-free egg replacer)

⅔ cup soymilk (or your choice of nondairy milk, plain or vanilla)

½ teaspoon ground cinnamon

½ teaspoon ground nutmeg

1 teaspoon pure vanilla extract

Vegetable oil, as desired for griddle

6 slices of whole-wheat bread

Powdered sugar

Maple syrup

Sliced kiwi fruit and strawberry halves for garnish (optional)

1 Whisk together the eggs, soymilk, spices, and vanilla.

2 Generously oil a griddle with 3 or 4 tablespoons of vegetable oil and heat it until a drop of water spatters when flicked onto the pan.

3 Dip both sides of each slice of bread into the soymilk mixture and transfer each slice to the heated griddle. The first side will take about 2 to 3 minutes to brown. Cook the second side for another 2 to 3 minutes, or until golden brown.

4 Remove the French toast from the griddle and place it on a serving plate. Dust each slice of French toast with powdered sugar and serve with a pitcher of warm maple syrup. If desired, garnish with thin slices of kiwi fruit and strawberry halves.

Vary It! *You can omit the eggs in this recipe if you simply add a tablespoon of flour to the soymilk mixture. Also, add a little more cinnamon or nutmeg to the powdered sugar if you would like a stronger flavor.*

Per serving: *Calories 315 (104 from Fat); Fat 12g (Saturated 2g); Cholesterol 2mg; Sodium 346mg; Carbohydrate 44g (Dietary Fiber 5g); Protein 11g.*

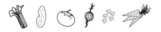

Chapter 10

Spectacular Soups, Salads, and Sides

In This Chapter

▶ Stirring up favorite soups

▶ Tossing some special salads

▶ Adding dairy-free extras

Soups, salads, and sides round out meals and contribute the color, flavor, texture, and temperature variety that add interest to meals. Of course, these foods don't necessarily have to play a support role at the table. Scale up the portion size of any of these foods, and they also can serve as the main course.

The recipes I include in this chapter represent a sample of several soups, salads, and sides likely to appeal to a range of palates. I include dairy-free versions of such classics as cream of tomato soup and cole slaw. For the more adventurous, I also include a delicious, traditional West African peanut-based soup.

Beginning with Soup

What better way to start a dinner or create an entire lunch than with some soup? A bowl of hot, steamy soup nourishes while it warms your toes. Soup also is a good way to work a few servings of vegetables and health-supporting fiber into your diet. And you can do it without dairy!

Although cream soups often are made with milk, cheese, and other dairy products, the soups in this collection aren't. The recipes I include in this section are thick, creamy, and hearty. The creaminess in these soups comes from non-dairy milk or cheese substitutes as well as white potatoes and sweet potatoes, which each lend their thickening power without the help of dairy products.

To add a creamy consistency to soups without using dairy products, purée about one-fourth of the batch of soup, including some veggies and broth, in a blender or food processor. (Chapter 8 provides information on these appliances.) Stir the puréed soup back into the larger batch and heat thoroughly. Adding beans, barley, rice, and small bits of pasta also thickens soups because these foods absorb some of the liquid.

Double any of the soup recipes that follow. Freeze leftovers and reheat them for lunches or dinner when you don't have time to cook. Making extra soup at home — and keeping the salt content low — instead of relying on canned soup can help you limit your sodium intake.

Broccoli and Cheddar Soup

Serve this hearty soup with a chunk of crusty bread. Add a small dish of fresh fruit salad for a cool and refreshing accompaniment. For maximum creaminess, I prefer to use plain soymilk or almond milk rather than rice milk or "light" varieties.

Preparation time: *10 minutes*

Cooking time: *About 45 minutes*

Yield: *6 entree-size servings*

3 tablespoons olive oil

1 medium yellow or white onion, chopped

2 to 3 cloves of garlic, chopped

4 cups vegetable or chicken broth

2 medium potatoes, peeled and cubed

2 cups plain soymilk or almond milk

12 ounces cheddar-style nondairy cheese, grated

One 10-ounce bag frozen, chopped broccoli florets or 1½ cups chopped, fresh broccoli florets

Freshly cracked black pepper

1 In a medium soup pot, heat olive oil. Add onions and garlic and cook over medium heat, stirring until onions become translucent, about 3 to 4 minutes.

2 Add broth and potatoes. Simmer with the lid on over medium heat for about 30 minutes.

3 When the soup is finished simmering, break up the potato pieces with a fork or potato masher. Add the soymilk or almond milk, cheese, and broccoli. Stir until the cheese is melted, cooking over low heat for about 15 minutes.

4 Add cracked black pepper to taste and serve.

Per serving: *Calories 289 (134 from Fat); Fat 15g (Saturated 1g); Cholesterol 0mg; Sodium 999mg; Carbohydrate 18g (Dietary Fiber 4g); Protein 20g.*

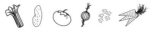

West African Peanut Soup

A good friend in Ghana shared this recipe with me years ago. This delicious African soup is traditionally served for celebrations and special occasions and works well for a North American Thanksgiving or wintertime event. It's rich and creamy with an intense peanut flavor.

Preparation time: *15 minutes*

Cooking time: *30 minutes*

Yield: *6 entree-size servings*

1 tablespoon olive oil

1 medium onion, chopped

1 teaspoon ground cumin

1 pound sweet potatoes, peeled, cooked, and cubed (or one 15-ounce can)

1 medium tart apple (such as Granny Smith), peeled and cubed

4 cups vegetable or chicken broth

⅛ teaspoon cinnamon

½ teaspoon black pepper

¼ cup creamy peanut butter

Nondairy sour cream or yogurt, for garnish

Chopped green onion or chives, for garnish

1 Heat the oil in a large saucepan. Add the onion and cumin and cook over medium heat, stirring frequently, until the onion is translucent, about 5 minutes.

2 Add the sweet potatoes, apple, broth, cinnamon, and black pepper and continue cooking over medium heat until the mixture boils, about 4 minutes.

3 Reduce the heat and simmer with the lid on for 20 to 30 minutes, or until the apples and vegetables are soft.

4 Stir in the peanut butter. Carefully transfer the hot soup to a blender and purée until smooth. (Because this soup is meant to be consistently creamy, purée the whole batch.) Alternatively, you can use an *immersion blender* to purée the soup. Directly place an immersion blender into the liquid ingredients to whip them without removing them from the pot.

5 Reheat the soup as needed after processing so that it's served piping hot. Garnish with a dollop of nondairy sour cream or nondairy plain yogurt and chopped green onions or chives.

Vary It! *For thinner soup, add more broth in Step 2. You also can replace the sweet potatoes and apple with white potatoes and carrots in approximately the same amounts (omit the cinnamon if you do so).*

Per serving: *Calories 186 (76 from Fat); Fat 8g (Saturated 2g); Cholesterol 0mg; Sodium 365mg; Carbohydrate 25g (Dietary Fiber 3g); Protein 5g.*

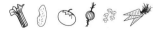

Cream of Tomato Soup

We called it Valentine soup when I was a child because as kids we thought tomato soup sounded yucky. Now it's a favorite, especially when it's homemade. Cream of tomato soup is an American classic when it's paired with a grilled (nondairy) cheese sandwich (see Chapter 11) and a crisp, tossed salad.

Preparation time: *10 minutes*

Cooking time: *About 45 minutes*

Yield: *6 entree-size servings*

4 tablespoons olive oil

Half a medium onion or one whole, small onion, diced

Two 15-ounce cans crushed tomatoes or 8 large, ripe tomatoes, chopped

4 tablespoons all-purpose flour

4 cups plain soymilk or almond milk

1 bay leaf

2 teaspoons sugar

1 teaspoon salt

1 In a small saucepan, heat 2 tablespoons of the olive oil. Add onions and cook over medium-high heat, stirring until onions become translucent, about 3 minutes.

2 Add the tomatoes and cook, uncovered, over medium heat for about 30 minutes.

3 Transfer the tomato mixture to a blender and purée until the mixture is smooth. Strain the mixture by passing it through a stainless steel sieve. Set aside.

4 In a medium saucepan, heat the remaining olive oil and stir in the flour. Add the milk, bay leaf, sugar, and salt. Cook over medium-high heat, stirring constantly, until the mixture begins to simmer, about 10 minutes.

5 Slowly add the strained tomato mixture to the milk mixture, stirring to blend. Bring the soup back to a simmer. Discard bay leaf and serve hot.

Per serving: Calories 214 (110 from Fat); Fat 12g (Saturated 2g); Cholesterol 0mg; Sodium 850mg; Carbohydrate 20g (Dietary Fiber 4g); Protein 8g.

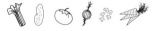

Creamy Potato and Leek Soup

Leeks, which look like large green onions or scallions, have a delicate, slightly sweet flavor that complements but doesn't overpower the mild flavor of potatoes. Pair this soup with the Roasted Red Pepper and Cheese Panini (see Chapter 11) and a tossed green salad.

Preparation time: *20 minutes*

Cooking time: *45 to 50 minutes*

Yield: *4 large servings*

¼ cup olive oil	32 ounces vegetable or chicken broth
4 large leeks, white and light green parts only	Salt and pepper to taste
2 large white potatoes (about 1 pound total), peeled and cubed	

1 In a medium saucepan, heat the olive oil. Wash the leeks well before cooking. Quarter the leeks and slice thinly (check out Figure 10-1 for help). Add the leeks to the saucepan, cover, and cook over medium heat until softened, about 8 minutes. Stir occasionally to prevent sticking.

2 Add potatoes and broth. Bring the mixture to a simmer over medium-high heat (about 10 minutes). Cover, lower heat to medium, and cook for another 30 minutes, or until potatoes are soft. Stir occasionally to prevent sticking.

3 Transfer the mixture to a blender or use an immersion blender to purée until smooth. Reheat and add salt and pepper to taste. Serve hot.

Per serving: Calories 265 (129 from Fat); Fat 14g (Saturated 2g); Cholesterol 0mg; Sodium 594mg; Carbohydrate 32g (Dietary Fiber 4g); Protein 4g.

HOW TO SLICE LEEKS

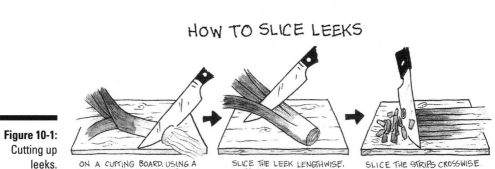

Figure 10-1: Cutting up leeks.

ON A CUTTING BOARD, USING A CHEF'S KNIFE, CUT OFF THE ROOT ENDS OF THE LEEKS.

SLICE THE LEEK LENGTHWISE, WITH THE TIP OF THE KNIFE.

SLICE THE STRIPS CROSSWISE INTO SMALL PIECES.

Serving Up Some Salad

Salads are a great way to add some crunchy vegetables to your diet. They also have many uses. You can serve a scoop of salad with a sandwich as a nice side, or you can let a big bowl of greens stand alone as a light lunch. What's even better: Salads are so versatile. If you have some fresh romaine or spinach, you can add different ingredients (all dairy-free) like in Figure 10-2 to infuse a little excitement to an otherwise plain salad.

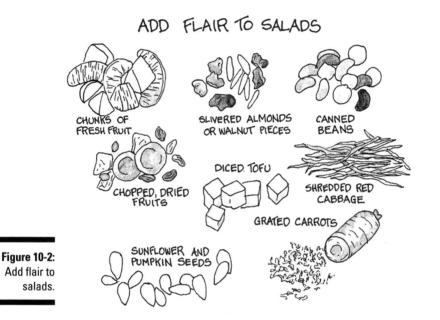

ADD FLAIR TO SALADS

CHUNKS OF FRESH FRUIT

SLIVERED ALMONDS OR WALNUT PIECES

CANNED BEANS

CHOPPED, DRIED FRUITS

DICED TOFU

SHREDDED RED CABBAGE

GRATED CARROTS

SUNFLOWER AND PUMPKIN SEEDS

Figure 10-2:
Add flair to
salads.

The first two salads I include in this section are tossed with creamy dressings you may think include dairy — but they don't. The last recipe is a tangy, vinaigrette-style slaw.

Mayonnaise generally doesn't contain dairy ingredients, but salads made with mayonnaise-based dressings sometimes contain milk added to thin the consistency of the dressing. If you go out to eat and order potato salad, tuna salad, carrot-raisin salad, or another salad made with a creamy dressing, ask whether dairy products were added.

Curried Carrot Raisin Salad

You may be familiar with traditional carrot raisin salad. The addition of curry powder, cumin, and allspice to this recipe spice up this version and give it a unique and delicious flavor. This salad is one of those dishes that's even better the next day. It keeps well in the refrigerator for several days.

Preparation time: *10 minutes*

Chill time: *1 hour, or overnight*

Yield: *6 servings*

3 cups peeled and grated carrots (about 6 medium carrots)

¼ cup light mayonnaise

1 cup raisins

⅓ cup crushed pineapple, drained

2 teaspoons curry powder

½ teaspoon ground cumin

¼ teaspoon ground allspice

Ground black pepper to taste

1 Place all ingredients in a medium mixing bowl. Toss well.

2 Chill for at least 1 hour before serving, or overnight for best flavor. Toss again before serving.

Vary It! *Add a handful of diced cooked chicken (or a soy-based chicken alternative) and stuff the mixture into a pita pocket for a sandwich.*

Per serving: *Calories150 (34 from Fat); Fat 4g (Saturated 1g); Cholesterol 3mg; Sodium 108mg; Carbohydrate 31g (Dietary Fiber 4g); Protein 1g.*

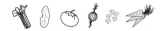

No-Dairy Waldorf Salad

The Waldorf salad you probably know makes an appearance around holiday time each year. The traditional style includes diced red apples, red grapes, chopped walnuts, celery, and lots of mayo. Some versions contain whipped cream or sour cream. This one is different. A light dressing made with soy yogurt or light mayonnaise and lemon juice adds just enough moisture, and the curry powder gives it some pizzazz. A nutritious comfort food you can dig in to! The salad will keep for three to five days in the refrigerator.

Preparation time: *About 15 minutes*

Chilling time: *2 hours*

Yield: *4 servings*

⅓ cup plain soy yogurt (or light mayonnaise)

⅓ cup light mayonnaise

2 tablespoons lemon juice

1 teaspoon lemon zest

2 teaspoons curry powder

½ teaspoon sugar

1 rib celery, diced (about ½ cup)

¾ cup seedless red grapes, halved

1 unpeeled, medium Granny Smith apple, diced

½ cup chopped walnuts

6 cups chopped Romaine lettuce

1 In a small bowl, whisk together yogurt, mayonnaise, lemon juice, zest, curry, and sugar to make the dressing.

2 In a large bowl, combine celery, grapes, apple, walnuts, and half of the dressing. Toss well using a flexible spatula or wooden spoon.

3 Add lettuce and remaining dressing. Toss to combine.

4 Chill for at least 2 hours and serve.

Vary It! *For a change of pace — a different flavor and slightly different look — add 3 tablespoons orange juice and ½ teaspoon powdered ginger in Step 1.*

Per serving: *Calories 235 (155 from Fat); Fat 17g (Saturated 2g); Cholesterol 7mg; Sodium 182mg; Carbohydrate 20g (Dietary Fiber 4g); Protein 5g.*

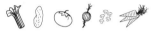

Confetti Cole Slaw

Cole slaw is a staple at any picnic or potluck dinner, although some are a tad on the boring side made with dairy. Why not add flair to your slaw and surprise everyone while keeping it dairy-free? Fresh ginger, rice vinegar, and red pepper flakes give this nutrient-packed slaw an extra kick. This salad will keep in the refrigerator for five to seven days.

Preparation time: *10 minutes*

Chilling time: *At least 2 hours*

Yield: *6 servings*

4 cups finely shredded cabbage (Combinations of green and red or purple cabbage are nice if you can find them.)

2 carrots, finely shredded

4 radishes, minced

½ cup chopped sweet onion

½ cup chopped green bell pepper (see Figure 10-3 for instruction)

2 cloves garlic, minced

¼ cup rice vinegar

1 tablespoon lemon juice

2 teaspoons sesame oil

1 teaspoon peeled and grated fresh ginger

1 teaspoon sesame seeds

½ teaspoon red pepper flakes

¼ teaspoon salt

Combine all the ingredients in a large bowl and toss well. Chill for at least 2 hours before serving. Toss again before serving.

Per serving: Calories 52 (17 from Fat); Fat 2g (Saturated 0g); Cholesterol 0mg; Sodium 121mg; Carbohydrate 8g (Dietary Fiber 3g); Protein 2g.

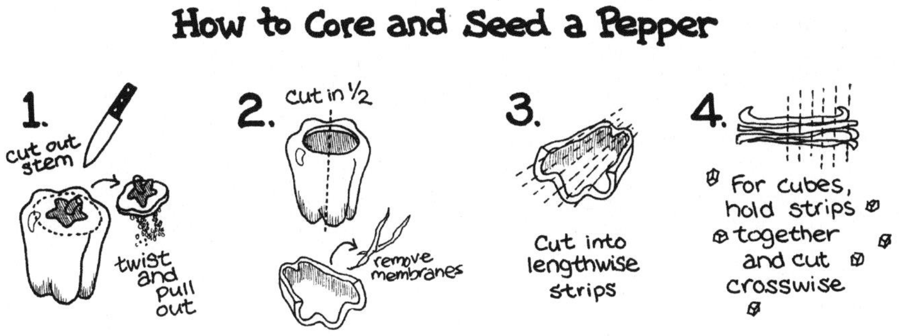

How to Core and Seed a Pepper

Figure 10-3: Coring, seeding, and chopping a green pepper.

1. cut out stem / twist and pull out

2. cut in ½ / remove membranes

3. Cut into lengthwise strips

4. For cubes, hold strips together and cut crosswise

Complementing Your Meal with Savory Sides

Although appetizers can set the tone for a meal and desserts can satisfy your sweet tooth, side dishes also are an important part to any meal. They round out your main dish. Even better, side dishes are a great way to add taste and comfort in smaller portions. The recipes in this section prove that creamy and cheesy comfort foods can still be yours to enjoy — dairy-free!

The classic mashed potatoes and gravy are simple to make and are indistinguishable in flavor from those made with cow's milk. The Stuffed Zucchini Boats work well as an accompaniment to a grilled sandwich or casserole (see Chapter 11). Or you can double the portion size and serve them as the main course.

As for the mac and cheese — you be the judge. In this version, I use soy cheddar-style cheese for its superior melt-ability. *Note:* Soy cheese may contain casein — check the ingredient label and pick a different cheese if you can't or don't want to eat casein. You can serve the dish as a side, but you'll probably like this recipe well enough to make it the main dish.

Creamed Potatoes with Brown Gravy

You may love mashed potatoes and gravy but have had to stay away from them in order to live dairy-free. Not anymore. These mashed potatoes are creamy and thick without the dairy products. Serve them with or without the dairy-free mushroom gravy shown here. Gravy lovers may want to double the gravy recipe to make sure there's enough to go around. Feel free to experiment with different potatoes until you find the one you like (see Figure 10-4).

Preparation time: *15 minutes*

Cooking time: *30 minutes*

Yield: *10 hefty servings of mashed potatoes and about 1½ cups of gravy*

Creamed Potatoes

5 pounds white potatoes, peeled and cut into 2-inch chunks (or halved if they're small)

¼ cup melted dairy-free, trans-fat-free margarine

1 cup plain almond milk (or your choice of plain nondairy milk)

¼ teaspoon salt

¼ teaspoon black pepper

1 Place the potatoes in a large pot and cover with cold water. Cook, covered, over medium-high heat until boiling. Reduce the heat, tilt the cover to allow steam to escape, and simmer for 30 minutes, or until the potatoes are tender. Drain.

2 In a large bowl, combine the potatoes, margarine, almond milk, salt, and pepper. Mash with a potato masher (or beat with a hand-mixer) until smooth and well blended. Use a wooden spoon to help blend the ingredients, if necessary. Transfer to a serving dish and serve with Mushroom Gravy (see the following recipe).

Tip: Start the gravy (see the following recipe) while your potatoes are cooking, and your meal will come together without a rush.

Brown Gravy

1 tablespoon olive oil

1 pound fresh mushrooms, thinly sliced

1 medium yellow or white onion, chopped

2 tablespoons flour

1 vegetable or chicken bouillon cube

¼ teaspoon salt (if using a sodium-free bouillon cube; otherwise omit)

¼ teaspoon black pepper

1 cup plain soymilk (or your choice of plain nondairy milk)

1 Heat the olive oil in a medium skillet. Add the mushrooms and onion and cook until the onion is translucent, about 5 minutes.

2 Add the flour and crumble the bouillon cube into the skillet. Add the salt (if needed) and pepper and stir.

3 Add the soymilk. Cook and stir for 2 to 3 minutes, until the gravy thickens and the ingredients are well blended. Pour into a bowl with a small ladle or large serving spoon and serve with Creamed Potatoes (see preceding recipe).

Tip: If you don't serve the gravy immediately, it may need to be reheated in a microwave, or you can hold it on the stovetop, warming, until ready to eat.

Per serving: *Calories 257 (63 from Fat); Fat 7g (Saturated 2g); Cholesterol 0mg; Sodium 246mg; Carbohydrate 44g (Dietary Fiber 5g); Protein 6g.*

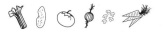

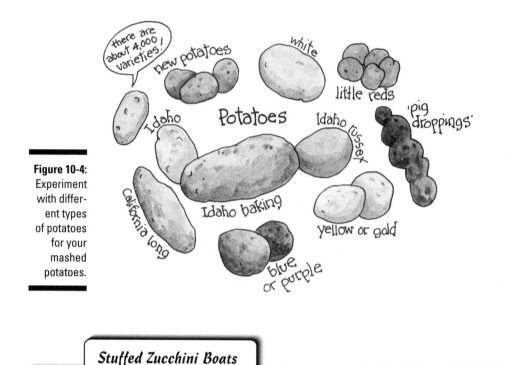

Figure 10-4:
Experiment with different ent types of potatoes for your mashed potatoes.

Stuffed Zucchini Boats

This recipe is adapted from an old favorite from the *Moosewood Cookbook* by Mollie Katzen. Nondairy Swiss-style cheese is mixed into the filling where the hot, moist ingredients help it to melt. This dish is a fun and tasty way to get your veggies, too.

Preparation time: *About 40 minutes*

Cooking time: *30 to 40 minutes*

Yield: *8 servings as sides, or 4 if served as the entree*

4 medium zucchini	*½ pound fresh mushrooms, diced*
2 tablespoons olive oil	*6 cloves of garlic, minced*
1½ cups chopped yellow or white onion	*1½ cups cooked rice (brown or white)*
1 teaspoon salt	*1½ cups ground almonds*

6 ounces Swiss-style nondairy cheese, grated

3 tablespoons lemon juice

Black pepper and cayenne pepper

Small handful of freshly minced herbs
(parsley, basil, thyme, dill, chives, marjoram), if

desired (If fresh herbs aren't available, use ½
to 1 teaspoon each of dried herbs.) (Refer to
Figure 10-5.)

Paprika

1 Cut each zucchini lengthwise down the middle. Cut a thin, flat layer on the bottom of each "boat" to help it lie flat in the pan. Use a spoon to scoop out the pulp, leaving boats with ¼-inch shells. Finely mince the pulp, and set aside the boats. Preheat the oven to 350 degrees.

2 Heat the olive oil in a medium-sized skillet. Add the onion and salt, and sauté over medium heat for 5 to 8 minutes, or until the onion is soft and translucent.

3 Add the zucchini pulp and mushrooms, and sauté another 8 to 10 minutes. Add the garlic during the last few minutes, stirring often to avoid browning it.

4 Place the rice and almonds in a medium-sized bowl. Stir in the sautéed mixture, all but about 2 ounces of grated cheese, and lemon juice and mix well. Season to taste with black pepper, cayenne pepper, and the fresh herbs (if desired).

5 Stuff the zucchini boats with the filling mixture. Sprinkle the tops with remaining cheese, and then add a dash of paprika for color. Place the boats in an oiled 9-x-13-inch baking dish, and bake for 30 to 40 minutes, or until heated through. Serve hot.

Vary It! Add ½ pound precooked ground turkey or soy sausage crumbles in Step 3. You also can substitute cooked quinoa, couscous, or another grain for the rice for a change of pace.

Per serving: Calories 249 (137 from Fat); Fat 15g (Saturated 1g); Cholesterol 0mg; Sodium 298mg; Carbohydrate 21g (Dietary Fiber 5g); Protein 12g.

Mincing Parsley & Other Fresh Herbs

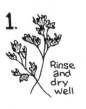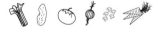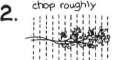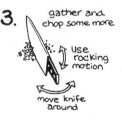

Figure 10-5: How to mince parsley and other fresh herbs.

1. Rinse and dry well

2. chop roughly
*NOTE: For herbs like rosemary and thyme, remove and chop leaves. Discard thick stem.

3. gather and chop some more / use rocking motion / move knife around

Macaroni and Cheese

Making macaroni and cheese from scratch takes about the same amount of time as it does to make it from a packaged mix. Homemade tastes better, and you can add variety by using different-shaped pasta noodles, including bow tie, elbow macaroni, penne, and small shells. This nondairy version looks and tastes very similar to traditional recipes. Soy cheese works best for this recipe (because of its melting quality), but some varieties contain casein. If you can't use it, try using nondairy pepper jack or American-style cheese.

Cooking time: *About 20 minutes*

Yield: *8 servings*

½ cup dairy-free, trans-fat-free margarine

½ cup flour

½ teaspoon salt

4 cups soymilk (or your choice of plain nondairy milk)

12 ounces cheddar-style soy cheese, grated (Caution: Cheddar-style soy cheese may contain casein, so read the label.)

16 ounces small whole-wheat pasta

Freshly cracked black pepper

1 In a small saucepan, melt the margarine over low heat, and then add the flour and salt. Cook for about 2 minutes, stirring constantly as mixture bubbles.

2 Slowly stir in the soymilk, and then add the cheese. Cook over medium-high heat until the mixture begins to boil, about 6 minutes. Stir constantly to keep soy cheese blended. Remove from heat.

3 In a large saucepan, bring 8 cups of water to a boil. Add pasta and cook for 8 minutes. Drain. (To save time, you can cook the pasta while the cheese sauce is cooking. Or you can have cooked noodles on hand and reheat them in the microwave.)

4 Add the cheese sauce to the hot pasta and toss well with a wooden spoon. Serve with lots of freshly cracked black pepper.

Vary It! *Add a 15-ounce can of stewed tomatoes in Step 4 for a change of pace and to add color to this dish. A dash of cayenne pepper also is good. Another option: Spoon the mac and cheese into an oiled baking dish and sprinkle some bread crumbs on top. Pop it into the oven and bake for 20 to 30 minutes at 350 degrees, or until top is golden brown.*

Per serving: Calories 458 (169 from Fat); Fat 19g (Saturated 5g); Cholesterol 0mg; Sodium 786mg; Carbohydrate 51g (Dietary Fiber 7g); Protein 23g.

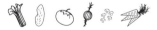

Chapter 11

Delectable Main Dishes

In This Chapter

- Transforming classics
- Working with sandwiches
- Experimenting with ethnic options

Your entree is the foundation of the dining experience. If the entree tastes good, you'll remember that meal for a while, and it may become part of your collection of family favorites. Now's the time to begin to compile your own main dish starting line-up.

Eliminating dairy from your favorite entrees may be somewhat challenging. Some entrees are dairy-free without even trying, such as stir-fry over rice or spaghetti with tomato sauce, for instance. They don't have any dairy in them unless you reach for a glass of milk or the Parmesan cheese shaker. On the other hand, however, many entree recipes do contain a lot of dairy as a result of North Americans' love for cheese and other dairy products. Think about some of your favorite comfort foods like grilled cheese sandwiches, creamy casseroles, and lasagna smothered in cheese.

The sampling of recipes I share in this chapter includes a mix of recipes that are dairy-free from the start as well as those that require you to swap dairy ingredients with nondairy alternatives. A couple of them are fairly simple; I include them to show you how to make classics dairy-free.

Because entrees make up a sizable portion of your diet, in this chapter I also aim for recipes to be generally aligned with advice for an eating style that promotes health. The recipes encourage heavier use of fruits, vegetables, and whole grains, and they discourage dependence on meat, sodium, saturated fat, trans fat, and added sugars.

Creating Some Hearty Family Favorites

The recipes in this section definitely fall into the category of comfort foods. They're foods that everyone likes; they're warm, creamy, easy-to-eat, stick-to-your ribs dishes that go well with a big chunk of good bread and a green salad on a chilly evening.

Just because you're eliminating dairy from your diet doesn't mean you have to change your love for these types of creamy comfort dishes. All you have to do is use your newfound dairy-free cooking skills and a few secret ingredients — nondairy alternatives — to replace the dairy in the traditional recipes. The examples in this section demonstrate how tasty the results can be.

Manicotti and many other pasta dishes freeze well. Consider making a double batch and freezing half. That way, you'll have a quick, dairy-free dinner (or lunch!) ready to reheat when you don't have time to cook from scratch.

Manicotti with Tofu, Spinach, and Mushrooms

Manicotti is a traditional Italian dish made with long, hollow tubes of pasta that are about 4 inches long and 1 inch in diameter. The pasta tubes are cooked and then filled with a mixture of cheese and herbs and topped with a tomato-based pasta sauce. In this version, tofu replaces the cheese, and nondairy Parmesan cheese replaces the dairy-based variety. The result is a rich, flavorful dish that's free of saturated fat and dairy ingredients.

Preparation time: *About 30 minutes*

Cooking time: *30 minutes*

Yield: *6 servings*

6 manicotti tubes

10-ounce package frozen chopped spinach, thawed, or 6 cups fresh spinach leaves

2 tablespoons olive oil

1 clove of garlic, minced

1 medium yellow or white onion, chopped

One 4-ounce can sliced mushrooms, drained and chopped (about 2 cups fresh, sliced)

16 ounces firm tofu

Juice of 1 lemon

1 teaspoon salt, if desired

½ teaspoon black pepper

2 cups spaghetti sauce (any bottled or fresh variety)

Soy Parmesan cheese

Chopped fresh, flat-leaf parsley and black olives for garnish

1 Preheat the oven to 350 degrees, and cook the manicotti according to the package directions. While the pasta cooks, drain the chopped spinach and squeeze out any remaining water. Set aside.

2 In a large skillet, heat the olive oil. Cook the garlic and onion in the oil over medium heat until the onions are translucent, about 10 minutes. Add the mushrooms to the onion mixture. Sauté for an additional minute. Add the spinach to the onion mixture and sauté over low heat for 1 to 2 minutes, turning the contents of the skillet with a spatula to help combine them. Remove from the heat and set aside.

3 In a large bowl, place the tofu, lemon juice, salt, and black pepper. Mash well with a potato masher or fork. Add the contents of the skillet to the tofu mixture. Mix well, using your hands if necessary to combine the ingredients thoroughly.

4 Oil a medium-sized rectangular baking pan or decorative casserole dish. Spoon two or three scoops of spaghetti sauce (about ½ cup) onto the bottom of the pan and spread evenly.

5 Fill each manicotti tube with some of the tofu mixture. (Portioning the filling first may help so you don't come up short when you get to the last couple of manicotti.) Place the manicotti side by side in the baking dish and cover with the remaining tomato sauce. (If you have extra tofu mixture left over, you can mix some of it into the tomato sauce before pouring it over the top of the manicotti.) Sprinkle the tops of the manicotti lightly with soy Parmesan cheese.

6 Cover the pan loosely with aluminum foil and bake for 30 minutes. Remove the foil for the last 10 minutes of baking time. Before serving, scatter chopped parsley and black olives over the top to garnish.

Vary It! *If manicotti tubes aren't available, you can substitute cooked lasagna noodles. Spread the filling on the noodles and roll them up instead of making filled tubes. You also can substitute chopped broccoli for the spinach if desired. Ramp up the flavor by adding your choice of several teaspoons of chopped, fresh herbs, such as oregano, basil, or thyme, to the filling.*

Per serving: *Calories 430 (124 from Fat); Fat 14g (Saturated 2g); Cholesterol 0mg; Sodium 450mg; Carbohydrate 58g (Dietary Fiber 7g); Protein 23g.*

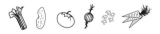

Chicken and Vegetable Casserole

Grated carrots and bits of red bell pepper add color, fiber, and a little sweetness to this delicious dish. Vegetarians can leave out the chicken or substitute soy-based veggie chicken.

Preparation time: *30 minutes*

Cooking time: *40 minutes*

Yield: *6 servings*

Chive Cream Sauce

4 tablespoons nondairy, trans-fat-free margarine

¼ cup plus 2 tablespoons all-purpose flour

½ teaspoon salt

½ teaspoon freshly ground black pepper

2 cups plain almond milk (or your choice of plain nondairy milk or soy creamer)

1 tablespoon minced fresh chives

1 In a small saucepan, melt the margarine and then whisk in the flour, salt, and pepper, stirring until smooth. Cook over medium heat for 3 to 5 minutes and then remove from the heat.

2 Gradually add the nondairy milk, stirring until smooth. Return the pan to the heat and cook, stirring constantly until thickened, about 10 minutes. Stir in chives and remove from the heat. Set aside.

Topping

2 tablespoons nondairy, trans-fat-free margarine

1 cup crushed stuffing mix (check ingredient list for dairy byproducts) or croutons

2 cups grated soy-based cheddar-style cheese

Combine margarine, stuffing mix, and soy cheese. Reserve 1 cup of this mixture for the topping and spread the remainder on the bottom of an oiled, oven-safe 2-quart casserole dish.

Filling

2 cups grated carrots

1½ cups sliced zucchini

1 cup chopped broccoli

1 cup fresh or frozen corn (see Figure 11-1 if you use fresh corn)

⅓ cup chopped yellow or white onion

½ cup chopped red bell pepper

6 ounces cooked, diced chicken or soy-based alternative

1 Preheat the oven to 350 degrees. Place vegetables in a bowl. Pour the Chive Cream Sauce (see earlier recipe) over the vegetables, add the chicken or soy substitute, and toss well to coat.

2 Spoon the filling into the prepared casserole dish, and then sprinkle with reserved topping (see preceding recipe). Casserole can be covered and refrigerated until ready to be baked. Bake, covered, for 40 minutes (10 minutes or so longer if the dish is taken from the refrigerator). Remove the cover for the last 10 minutes of baking. Casserole will be golden brown on top when done.

Vary It! *Other vegetables work well in this dish, too, including green peas, cauliflower, yellow squash, asparagus, and black olives.*

Per serving: *Calories 363 (178 from Fat); Fat 20g (Saturated 6g); Cholesterol 26mg; Sodium 1,026mg; Carbohydrate 29g (Dietary Fiber 6g); Protein 20g.*

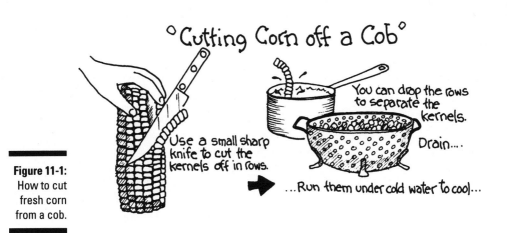

°Cutting Corn off a Cob°

Use a small sharp knife to cut the kernels off in rows.

You can drop the rows to separate the kernels.

Drain....

...Run them under cold water to cool...

Figure 11-1:
How to cut fresh corn from a cob.

Spaghetti with Spicy Marinara Sauce

This spicy, tangy pasta dish is sure to be a hit in your house. Using different shapes of pasta, including bow ties, shells, fettuccine, rotini, and others, can vary this simple dish.

Cooking time: *15 minutes*

Yield: *6 servings*

6 tablespoons olive oil

2 cloves of garlic, minced

½ teaspoon red pepper flakes

1 pound whole-wheat spaghetti

2 cups bottled or homemade marinara sauce (see Chapter 12 for a recipe)

¼ cup green olives, chopped

2 tablespoons capers, rinsed, drained, and minced

¼ cup flat-leaf parsley, chopped

1 teaspoon lemon zest

Nondairy Parmesan cheese to taste

Freshly ground black pepper to taste

Black olives and parsley for garnish

1 In a small skillet, add 2 tablespoons of olive oil and heat until hot but not smoking. Add garlic and red pepper flakes. Sauté over medium heat for 3 minutes and set aside.

2 In a large pot, cook the spaghetti according to the package instructions. Drain and set aside.

3 In a separate pot, heat tomato sauce until it just starts to boil.

4 In a large bowl, toss the pasta with the remaining olive oil, green olives, capers, parsley, and lemon zest. Next, add the marinara sauce and toss until well combined.

5 Serve on individual plates and add nondairy Parmesan cheese and freshly ground black pepper to taste. Garnish each plate with a black olive and a sprig of parsley.

Per serving: Calories 440 (145 from Fat); Fat 16g (Saturated 2g); Cholesterol 0mg; Sodium 386mg; Carbohydrate 66g (Dietary Fiber 11g); Protein 13g.

Easy Vegetable Lasagna

Tofu takes the place of ricotta cheese, adding protein while cutting the saturated fat, sodium, and lactose typically found in lasagna. Using plenty of spaghetti sauce keeps the dish moist and flavorful.

Preparation time: *35 minutes*

Cooking time: *1 hour*

Yield: *10 servings*

8 ounces whole-wheat lasagna noodles

1 tablespoon olive oil

1 large white or yellow onion, chopped

1 large head or 2 small heads broccoli, chopped into small pieces

2 medium zucchini, chopped into small pieces

24 ounces firm tofu

Juice of 1 lemon

4 egg whites (or equivalent amount of cholesterol-free egg white replacer)

1 teaspoon dried oregano

1 teaspoon dried thyme

¼ teaspoon dried dill

2 tablespoons dried parsley

½ teaspoon freshly ground black pepper

¾ cup grated nondairy Parmesan cheese

25-ounce jar prepared spaghetti sauce (more if you want to serve extra on the side)

3 cups shredded nondairy mozzarella-style cheese

1 Preheat the oven to 350 degrees, and cook the lasagna noodles according to the package instructions. Separate the noodles, pat them dry, and then set them aside.

2 In a medium skillet, heat the olive oil. Cook the onions in the oil over medium heat until they're translucent, about 7 minutes. Add the broccoli and zucchini and sauté for 2 to 3 minutes to partially cook. Remove from the heat.

3 In a medium bowl, mix the tofu, lemon juice, egg whites, oregano, thyme, dill, parsley, and black pepper and half the nondairy Parmesan cheese.

4 In a lightly oiled 13-x-17-inch pan, layer the lasagna as follows: Put a thin layer of tomato sauce on the bottom of the pan. Lay 4 lasagna noodles (or the number needed to fit the pan in a single layer; cut the noodles if necessary to fit). Add a layer of the tofu mixture, and then half the vegetable mixture, followed by half the mozzarella-style nondairy cheese. Repeat the layers, ending with a little more tomato sauce and the remaining nondairy Parmesan cheese.

5 Bake, covered loosely with aluminum foil for 1 hour, or until brown and bubbly. Remove foil for the last 10 to 15 minutes of baking.

Vary It! *You can spread some sun-dried tomato pesto or basil pesto on top of the lasagna along with the tomato sauce (or mixed in with the tomato sauce) when assembling the dish (see Chapter 12 for a nondairy pesto sauce recipe). Meat-eaters can add about ½ cup of cooked ground turkey to the layers in Step 4; vegetarians may prefer a similar amount of soy burger crumbles to add flavor and texture to the dish.*

Tip: *In some stores, you can find no-boil varieties of lasagna noodles. Try those to save yourself some time. With this variety, you can place noodles uncooked into the pan.*

Per serving: *Calories 344 (121 from Fat); Fat 14g (Saturated 1g); Cholesterol 0mg; Sodium 798mg; Carbohydrate 32g (Dietary Fiber 10g); Protein 30g.*

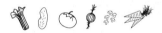

Zucchini Parmesan

This is a good dish to make in the summertime when gardens are full of zucchini squash and tomatoes. This is comfort food — rich, gooey, and full of flavor.

Preparation time: *30 minutes*

Cooking time: *30 minutes*

Yield: *4 servings*

4 large zucchini squash (about 2½ pounds)

¼ cup olive oil

3 or 4 large tomatoes (about ¾ pound), cored and seeded

¼ cup tomato paste

1 large egg (or equivalent amount of cholesterol-free egg replacer)

1 tablespoon chopped fresh flat-leaf parsley

Salt and pepper to taste

4 ounces nondairy mozzarella-style cheese, thinly sliced

½ cup grated nondairy Parmesan cheese

1 Preheat the oven to 300 degrees. Cut the zucchini into julienne strips, about 2 inches long and ¼ inch wide. Pat dry and set aside.

2 In a medium skillet, heat the olive oil over medium heat until the oil is hot but not smoking, about 4 minutes.

3 Transfer the zucchini strips to the skillet and pan-fry for 3 to 5 minutes. Remove the zucchini and set the strips on paper towel to absorb excess oil.

4 Combine the tomatoes, tomato paste, egg, parsley, salt, and pepper in a food processor or blender and process until smooth, about 2 minutes.

5 Coat an 8-x-8-inch glass baking dish or a quiche dish with vegetable spray. Pour about one-quarter of the tomato mixture into the pan and spread it evenly across the bottom. Arrange a quarter of the zucchini on top and then add a quarter of the nondairy mozzarella-style cheese and nondairy Parmesan cheese. Repeat the layers, ending with nondairy Parmesan cheese on top.

6 Bake uncovered for 30 minutes until brown and bubbly.

Vary It! *To get even more vegetables into your diet, mix zucchini and yellow squash, or add a handful of steamed and chopped carrots, broccoli, and cauliflower as you assemble the layers in Step 5.*

Per serving: Calories 338 (174 From Fat); Fat 19g (Saturated 2g); Cholesterol 53mg; Sodium 199mg; Carbohydrate 25g (Dietary Fiber 10g); Protein 23g.

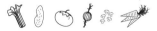

Sinking Your Teeth into Sandwiches

Hot sandwiches have a common ingredient that works like glue to help the fillings and bread stay together. That ingredient — you guessed it — is cheese . . . warm, stretchy, melted cheese.

The good news is that just because you're going dairy-free doesn't mean you have to avoid cheesy sandwiches. Many nondairy variations of cheddar, American, mozzarella, jack, Swiss, and others are available. Experiment with them to recreate your favorite cheesy sandwiches, such as the following, among others:

- ✔ **The Reuben:** I make mine with sauerkraut, nondairy Swiss cheese, and rye — no meat. Thousand Island dressing is a great addition if you like the taste. (Just be sure the brand you buy doesn't contain milk. Read the ingredient label to find out.)

- ✔ **The patty melt:** Try using a veggie burger patty and nondairy Swiss cheese. Add your favorite burger toppings (ketchup, a pickle, a scoop of salsa), as desired.

- ✔ **The grilled cheese-and-veggie:** One nice variation uses nondairy mozzarella cheese, roasted red peppers, and spinach.

In this section, I include two variations of the classic grilled cheese sandwich as well as the Mexican equivalent — the quesadilla!

Soy cheese works well in these sandwiches because it melts so well. However, if you use it, be aware that some brands contain casein, a milk protein, which you want to avoid if you're allergic to the milk protein.

Grilled Cheese and Tomato Sandwich

You don't have to avoid the classic grilled cheese just because you're eliminating dairy from your diet. This recipe recreates the famous sandwich with nondairy margarine and nondairy cheese. Serve it with Cream of Tomato Soup (Chapter 10) for a complete meal.

Cooking time: *10 minutes*

Yield: *2 servings*

4 slices of coarse whole-grain bread

2 tablespoons nondairy, trans-fat-free margarine

4 slices nondairy American-style cheese

One large, ripe tomato, sliced

Mayonnaise and a pickle spear, as desired

1 Heat a medium-sized cast-iron skillet (or other heavy skillet) over medium heat. Spread one side of each slice of bread with margarine.

2 Place two slices of bread, margarine side down, in the skillet. Layer two slices of cheese and a slice or two of tomato (arrange to fit) on each slice of bread. Top each sandwich with a second slice of bread, placed so that the margarine side faces up.

3 Cook on medium heat until the margarine melts and the bread browns, usually about 3 to 5 minutes (lift edges to check for doneness). When the first side of each sandwich is browned, use a spatula to flip each sandwich over. Continue cooking until the second side of each sandwich is browned and the cheese is melted, about 2 to 3 more minutes. Garnish with a dab of mayo and a pickle spear, if desired, and serve hot.

Tip: *When making grilled cheese sandwiches, the bread at times may brown before the cheese inside the sandwich has fully melted. If you see that happening, you can help the cheese along by covering the sandwich with the lid from a small saucepan. Just place the lid over the sandwich and continue to cook. After 1 minute, lift the lid and check to see whether the cheese has melted. Replace the lid and continue cooking as needed.*

Vary It! *Add extras to the filling, including roasted red peppers, alfalfa sprouts, or grilled onions, mushrooms, and red or yellow bell pepper strips. Or make your own signature version by adding a smear of Spinach and Basil Pesto Sauce (Chapter 12), sundried tomato pesto, black olive tapenade, honey mustard, or fruit chutney.*

Per serving: *Calories 319 (156 from Fat); Fat 17g (Saturated 5g); Cholesterol 0mg; Sodium 961mg; Carbohydrate 28g (Dietary Fiber 4g); Protein 14g.*

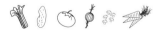

Roasted Red Pepper and Cheese Panini

A *panini* is an Italian-style sandwich grilled in a sandwich press, which often makes horizontal marks on the finished product. Panini presses are sold widely throughout North America and around the world. The roasted red pepper packs this version with flavor, and the nondairy cheese adds just the right amount of gooey cheesiness. Pair this sandwich with a cup of soup or a side of Confetti Cole Slaw (Chapter 10).

Preparation time: *10 minutes*

Cooking time: *10 minutes*

Yield: *2 servings*

Special equipment: *Panini press*

4 slices of thick, rustic-style bread, such as sourdough or Italian

4 tablespoons olive oil

4 slices of nondairy mozzarella-style cheese

Two large roasted red peppers packed in oil

Black olives (optional)

1 Use a pastry brush to liberally coat one side of each slice of bread with olive oil.

2 Place two slices of bread, oiled side down, on the bottom of the panini press. Layer two slices of cheese and one roasted red pepper (arrange to fit) on each slice of bread. Top each sandwich with a second slice of bread, placed so that the oiled side faces up.

3 Place the weighted top of the panini press on top of the sandwiches and cook on medium-high heat until the sandwich sizzles, the cheese melts, and the bread browns, about 5 minutes. When the sandwiches are done, remove the top press and use a spatula to lift sandwiches off the panini press. Serve hot with black olives (if desired).

Vary It! *Experiment with other fillings and spreads in Step 2. For example, add a smear of pesto sauce or mayonnaise, or add several fresh spinach leaves. Grilled onions also are good on this sandwich.*

Per serving: *Calories 828 (331 from Fat); Fat 37g (Saturated 5g); Cholesterol 0mg; Sodium 1,731mg; Carbohydrate 101g (Dietary Fiber 6g); Protein 25g.*

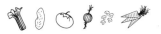

Vegetable and Cheese Quesadilla

These Mexican-style grilled "sandwiches" can be served as a main dish or cut into wedges and served as appetizers. Cheesy and full of flavor, they're a nice alternative to your mother's grilled cheese sandwich. Fruit slices on the side — or a dish of the Calypso Fruit Salad in Chapter 9 — make a refreshing accompaniment.

Preparation time: *5 minutes*

Cooking time: *About 25 minutes*

Yield: *2 servings*

2 cups of any mixture of grated carrots and chopped broccoli, onions, bell peppers, mushrooms, and asparagus

4 medium, whole-wheat flour tortillas

2 tablespoons nondairy, trans-fat-free margarine

1 cup grated nondairy cheddar-style cheese

Avocado slices, black olives, and nondairy sour cream (optional)

1 Place vegetables in a covered, microwave-safe dish with a few tablespoons of water. Steam the vegetables for 4 or 5 minutes, or until tender. Drain and set aside. Heat a medium-sized cast-iron skillet (or other heavy skillet) over medium heat.

2 Spread one side each of two tortillas with margarine. Place one tortilla, margarine side down, in the skillet. Layer ½ cup of the nondairy cheese and 1 cup of the steamed vegetables (arrange to fit) on the tortilla. Place the second tortilla, margarine side up, on top.

3 Cook over medium heat until margarine melts and the tortilla browns, about 4 or 5 minutes (lift edges after 3 minutes to check for doneness). When the first side of the quesadilla is browned, use a spatula to flip the quesadilla over. Continue cooking until the second side of the quesadilla is browned and the cheese is melted, about 3 minutes. Using a pizza cutter, slice the quesadilla into quarters, and then lift it from the skillet with a spatula and set aside.

4 Repeat Steps 2 and 3 to make a second quesadilla. Garnish the finished quesadillas with avocado slices, black olives, and a dollop of nondairy sour cream (if desired).

Tip: *Chop the vegetables into tiny pieces so that large chunks don't fall out when you flip the quesadilla.*

Vary It! *Add a handful of diced, cooked salmon or chicken or soy-based chicken chunks to each quesadilla.*

Per serving: *Calories 493 (192 from Fat); Fat 21g (Saturated 5g); Cholesterol 0mg; Sodium 1,102mg; Carbohydrate 56g (Dietary Fiber 10g); Protein 26g.*

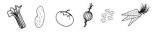

Enticing Your Palate with Ethnic Entrees

Dairy ingredients characterize many of the foods prepared in Northern and Northwestern Europe as well as in North America. In other parts of the world, though, these ingredients play a much smaller role — or none at all. If you're up for trying some different ethnic foods, going dairy-free doesn't have to be as dramatic a change as with most traditional entrees you may eat.

I hope the following recipes inspire you to experiment with other recipes from cultures outside your own. Your reward will be a much bigger collection of recipes to draw from as you plan meals. As you experiment with new foods, expect to find a few duds along the way, which is okay because you'll also find some new favorites, too.

The great thing about these recipes is that you won't have to shuttle around town trying to find unusual ingredients. You can find most of the ingredients in these recipes at your local grocery store.

Spicy Vegetable Curry

Curry is the word used to refer to spicy dishes unique to South Asian cooking. Curry powder, a mixture of savory spices, is a key ingredient. This traditional nondairy dish from India is rich in fiber and flavor. Control the "heat" to suit your own palate by increasing or decreasing the amount of chili powder you add.

Preparation time: *15 minutes*

Cooking time: *About 50 minutes*

Yield: *4 servings*

¼ cup olive oil

1 large white or yellow onion, chopped

2 cloves of garlic, minced

1 bay leaf

1 tablespoon ground coriander

1 tablespoon ground cumin

1 teaspoon ground ginger

1 teaspoon ground chili powder (or more to taste)

One 15-ounce can of stewed tomatoes or 4 large, ripe tomatoes

Freshly ground black pepper to taste

One 15-ounce can garbanzo beans (chickpeas), drained

1½ cups water

3 large carrots, thinly sliced

1 cup cauliflower florets, broken into smaller pieces

2 large potatoes, peeled and diced

1 cup fresh or frozen green peas

2 cups cooked brown rice

1 In a large saucepan, heat the olive oil. Add the onion, garlic, bay leaf, and spices, cooking over medium heat for about 10 minutes, or until the onion is translucent. Stir to prevent sticking.

2 Add the tomatoes, pepper, garbanzo beans, and water. Cook over medium heat, simmering for 10 minutes. Add the carrots, cauliflower, and potatoes and continue simmering over medium heat for another 20 minutes, or until the beans and vegetables are tender.

3 Add the peas and simmer for an additional 5 minutes. (If using frozen peas, let them simmer a few extra minutes to make sure they're heated thoroughly.) Remove from the heat and serve over rice.

Vary It! *Add 1 cup of diced, cooked chicken or a soy-based chicken alternative in Step 2.*

Per serving: Calories 528 (148 from Fat); Fat 16g (Saturated 2g); Cholesterol 0mg; Sodium 560mg; Carbohydrate 85g (Dietary Fiber 15g); Protein 13g.

Baked Seven-Layer Burritos

Burritos are a whole meal all wrapped up in a flour tortilla. The burritos I show here combine the great flavors and contrasting colors of beans, sweet potatoes, rice, cheese, salsa, and fresh veggies. You can assemble this dish the night before and have it ready to place into the oven the next day. Leftovers are great reheated. These are big — potentially messy — burritos, so plan to eat them with a knife and fork, rather than with your hands!

Preparation time: *10 minutes*

Cooking time: *10 minutes*

Yield: *4 burritos*

One 15-ounce can black beans, rinsed and drained

One 15-ounce can sweet potatoes (or about 2 cups fresh, cooked sweet potatoes)

Four 10-inch flour tortillas

2 cups cooked brown rice

2 cups salsa

½ cup grated nondairy cheddar-style cheese

1 cup chopped Romaine lettuce

1 large ripe tomato, cored, seeded, and diced

2 green onions, minced

4 black olives, chopped

1 small avocado, peeled and mashed

½ cup plain soy yogurt (optional)

1 Preheat the oven to 350 degrees. Heat the black beans in a small saucepan over low heat for about 5 minutes, or until steaming hot. In another small saucepan, heat the sweet potatoes. When steamy and heated through, mash them with a potato masher or fork and stir until smooth. Set both aside.

2 Lay each tortilla flat on a cutting board. Spoon about ⅓ cup of the sweet potatoes, ⅓ cup of beans, and ½ cup of rice onto the center of each tortilla.

3 Fold one end of a tortilla toward the middle, and then fold the sides toward the middle (check out Figure 11-2 for more on folding a burrito). Place the burrito into an oiled 8-x-8-inch baking dish. Make sure the end of the fold is tucked underneath so the burrito doesn't unroll. Repeat to make three more burritos, arranging them side by side in the baking dish.

4 Spoon the salsa evenly over the burritos. Top with the grated cheese. Cover the baking dish with foil and bake for 30 minutes, removing the foil for the last 10 minutes of baking. Remove the burritos from the oven when they're thoroughly heated and the cheese has melted.

5 Divide the remaining ingredients among the four burritos. Top each burrito with chopped lettuce, tomato, onions, black olives, avocado, and a dollop of soy yogurt (optional). Serve immediately.

Per serving: *Calories 697 (145 from Fat); Fat 16g (Saturated 3g); Cholesterol 0mg; Sodium 1,545mg; Carbohydrate 118g (Dietary Fiber 14g); Protein 23g.*

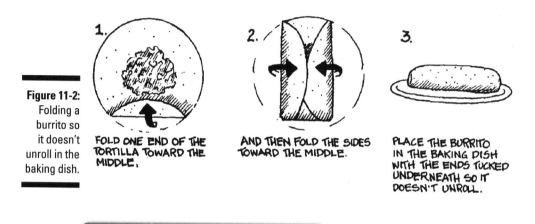

FOLDING A BURRITO

Figure 11-2:
Folding a burrito so it doesn't unroll in the baking dish.

1. FOLD ONE END OF THE TORTILLA TOWARD THE MIDDLE.

2. AND THEN FOLD THE SIDES TOWARD THE MIDDLE.

3. PLACE THE BURRITO IN THE BAKING DISH WITH THE ENDS TUCKED UNDERNEATH SO IT DOESN'T UNROLL.

Spanish Paella with Shrimp

Paella (pa YEY a) is a traditional, nondairy Spanish rice dish made with vegetables, olive oil, saffron, and tiny bits of fish or meat. There are many ways to make this dish, so you can create your own variations using your favorite ingredients. This version can get you started.

Preparation time: *15 minutes*

Cooking time: *About 65 minutes*

Yield: *4 servings*

¼ cup olive oil

2 large white or yellow onions, sliced

2 large cloves of garlic, minced

1½ cups uncooked brown rice

4 cups water or chicken stock

1½ teaspoons saffron

1 teaspoon salt

Freshly ground black pepper to taste

4 large carrots, thinly sliced

1 large red bell pepper, sliced

8 ounces deveined shrimp (optional; see Figure 11-3 for help)

Handful or two of soy-based sausage crumbles (optional)

4 tomatoes, peeled and diced

1 cup fresh or frozen green peas

Fresh lemon wedges for garnish

1 In a large saucepan, heat the olive oil. Add the onions and garlic, cooking over medium heat for about 10 minutes, or until onions are translucent. Stir to prevent sticking.

2 Add the rice, water or chicken stock, saffron, salt, and pepper. Cook over high heat until the water boils, and then cover and lower the heat to simmer for about 20 minutes.

3 Add the carrots and bell pepper. Simmer for an additional 20 minutes. Add the shrimp and sausage, if desired, for the last 10 minutes of cooking. Stirring isn't necessary. Add the tomatoes and peas.

4 Remove the saucepan from the heat, cover, and let everything set for 15 minutes, or until the remainder of the water is absorbed. Stir to mix the ingredients.

5 Place the saucepan back on the stovetop and reheat. Transfer to a serving dish and garnish with lemon wedges.

Vary It! *Add odd bits of vegetables that you may have on hand, including celery, leeks, yellow squash, zucchini, and others.*

Tip: *If you make paella often, consider investing in a paella pan, a heavy, flat-bottomed pan with handles on two sides. You can cook the paella and serve it from the same pan.*

Per serving: *Calories 546 (153 from Fat); Fat 17g (Saturated 3g); Cholesterol 84mg; Sodium 772mg; Carbohydrate 81g (Dietary Fiber 12g); Protein 20g.*

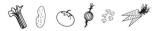

Cleaning and Deveining Shrimp

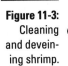

Figure 11-3:
Cleaning and deveining shrimp.

1.

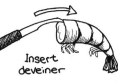

Insert deveiner

2.

Push toward the tail

vein

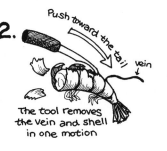

The tool removes the vein and shell in one motion

3.

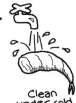

Clean under cold water

Indonesian Saté

Saté (pronounced "sah TAY") is a traditional Indonesian dish made with grilled meat, fish, or tofu and peanut sauce (I opt for tofu here). The peanut sauce has the consistency of a creamy, dairy-based sauce. Serve this dish with steamed vegetables and rice. If you use crunchy peanut butter, the tofu slices will be topped with ground nuts, which look nice and adds crunch. Marinating the tofu slices isn't necessary, but doing so lends a stronger flavor.

Preparation time: *15 minutes*

Marinating time: *2 hours*

Cooking time: *25 minutes*

Yield: *4 servings*

½ teaspoon cider vinegar	¼ cup reduced-sodium soy sauce
¼ cup peanut butter	¼ cup boiling water
1 tablespoon vegetable oil	⅛ teaspoon cayenne pepper
¼ teaspoon finely crumbled bay leaf	¼ teaspoon ground ginger
2 teaspoons honey	16 ounces firm tofu

1 Preheat the oven to 375 degrees. Lightly oil the bottom and sides of a 9-x-13-inch baking pan or shallow casserole dish and set aside.

2 In a small bowl or cup, whisk together the vinegar, peanut butter, oil, bay leaf, honey, soy sauce, water, cayenne pepper, and ginger, mixing well. (Alternatively, use a blender, which helps to break up the bay leaf, too.)

3 Spread a thin layer of the peanut butter mixture across the bottom of the prepared baking pan.

4 Slice the tofu into ½-inch slabs and lay flat, one layer thick, in the baking pan. Pour the remaining sauce evenly over the top of the tofu. If desired, marinate the tofu in the refrigerator for 2 hours.

5 Bake the tofu, uncovered, for 25 minutes. This dish is delicious served over rice noodles with steamed vegetables.

Vary It! *Substitute fish or chicken for tofu or use soy-based veggie alternatives.*

Per serving: *Calories 218 (133 from Fat); Fat 15g (Saturated 2g); Cholesterol 0mg; Sodium 721mg; Carbohydrate 10g (Dietary Fiber 1g); Protein 12g.*

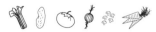

Chapter 12

Dairy-Free Dips, Spreads, Sauces, and Dressings

In This Chapter

▶ Creating delicious dips

▶ Discovering dairy-free spreads

▶ Cooking with flavorful sauces

▶ Dressing your salads without dairy

*Y*our imagination is all that stands between you and a vast collection of condiments that can add flavor and interest to meals. Homemade dips, spreads, sauces, and dressings taste extra good, because they're fresh. And because you make them yourself, you can easily leave out — or add — the ingredients you prefer.

Customizing your condiments makes it a cinch to create meals with all the flavor you want but without the dairy ingredients you want to avoid — and you can save money that way, too. Instead of paying premium prices for specialty products, such as those sold in natural foods stores, you can make your own for a fraction of the cost. The recipes I include in this chapter are quick and easy to make, and they use common ingredients you can find in most neighborhood supermarkets.

Try your hand at the examples I include here, and then let these recipes serve as your inspiration to make others on your own. Use the information in Chapter 8 to modify your favorite traditional recipes to be dairy-free and to create brand-new recipes of your own.

Drumming Up Some Divine Dips

A *dip* is a type of sauce used to add flavor to foods. Rather than being poured over the food, though, like other sauces, foods eaten with dips are, well, dipped into it. Foods eaten with dips usually are those you can hold in your hand. They're *finger foods,* such as carrots and other cut vegetables, crackers, bread sticks, tortilla chips, pita bread points, fruit slices, and others.

Dips commonly are made with sour cream, yogurt, or melted cheese as the base. The recipes I include here, though, either use nondairy substitutes or no dairy or dairy-like ingredients at all. In the recipes for Baba Ghanouj (pronounced ba-ba ga NOOSH) and Spinach and Artichoke Hummus — both traditional Middle Eastern foods — nothing but puréed vegetables or beans, *tahini* (sesame paste), and some spices are needed to create delicious creamy dips. The Bean and Cheese Dip recipe benefits from easy-to-melt, creamy soy cheddar-style cheese.

Baba Ghanouj

This naturally dairy-free Middle Eastern eggplant dip is delicious served with toasted pita points or crackers. It's also thick enough to be used as a spread on whole-wheat toast and as a sandwich filling.

Preparation time: *30 minutes (including time for the eggplant to cool after baking)*

Cooking time: *1 hour*

Chilling time: *1 hour*

Yield: *Six ¼-cup servings*

1 pound of eggplant (about 2 medium)	3 tablespoons lemon juice
3 tablespoons tahini	¼ cup finely chopped flat-leaf parsley
2 teaspoons minced garlic (see Figure 12-1)	

1 Preheat the oven to 350 degrees. Lightly grease a 9-x-13-inch baking pan.

2 Slice the eggplant in half lengthwise and place the halves in the baking pan, insides facing down. Cover the pan with foil.

3 Bake the eggplant for about 1 hour, or until soft. Remove it from the oven, take off the foil, and allow the eggplant to cool enough to be handled, about 15 minutes.

4 Scoop out the eggplant seeds with a spoon and discard, and then use a paring knife to gently peel off the outer dark skin. (It will be easy to remove. The eggplant flattens a lot, so it's easy to remove innards, too.) Discard seeds and skin.

5 Chop eggplant and place it in a blender or food processor. Add the remaining ingredients and blend until smooth. Using a spatula, transfer the mixture into a serving bowl. Chill for 1 hour before serving with warm pita wedges for dipping.

Tip: Tahini is a paste made from ground sesame seeds. It has a mild sesame flavor and is used as an ingredient in many dips, glazes, and salad dressings. You can find tahini at natural foods stores, Middle Eastern and specialty stores, and now many supermarkets. It's often sold in a can with a plastic lid or in a jar, like natural peanut butter, with a layer of oil floating on top. Stir in the oil before scooping out the tahini.

Per serving: Calories 67 (37 from Fat); Fat 4g (Saturated 1g); Cholesterol 0mg; Sodium 6mg; Carbohydrate 7g (Dietary Fiber 2g); Protein 2g.

Mincing garlic

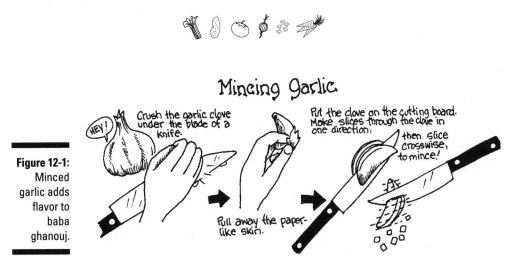

Figure 12-1: Minced garlic adds flavor to baba ghanouj.

Spinach and Artichoke Hummus

Hummus is a traditional Middle Eastern bean dip made with garbanzo beans (chickpeas), tahini, garlic, lemon juice, and spices. You can make endless variations by experimenting with other added ingredients. Ready-made hummus is expensive to buy, so save money and make your own at home quickly and easily.

Preparation time: *10 minutes*

Yield: *Six ½-cup servings*

One 15-ounce can garbanzo beans (chickpeas), rinsed and drained

¼ cup water

½ cup frozen, chopped spinach, thawed and well-drained, or about 2 cups of fresh leaves

1 large clove of garlic, minced

¼ cup tahini

¼ cup lemon juice

¼ teaspoon ground cumin

½ cup artichoke hearts (refer to Figure 12-2 for guidance)

2 teaspoons extra-virgin olive oil

Half a lemon

Paprika

1 Place the garbanzo beans, water, spinach, garlic, tahini, lemon juice, and cumin in a blender or food processor and process until smooth and creamy.

2 Add the artichoke hearts and pulse the blender or food processor a few times so that the artichoke hearts are chopped up but not quite puréed. Pour the dip into a shallow bowl.

3 Drizzle the olive oil over the hummus, followed by a squeeze of fresh lemon juice and a dusting of paprika. Chill if desired and then serve.

Vary It! *For a change of pace, replace spinach and artichokes with a roasted red bell pepper, several sun-dried tomatoes, ¼ cup sliced jalapeño peppers, or 1 tablespoon chopped fresh dill in Step 1. Any of these additions gives the dip a fundamentally different — and delicious — flavor.*

Per serving: Calories 127 (68 from Fat); Fat 8g (Saturated 1g); Cholesterol 0mg; Sodium 104mg; Carbohydrate 12g (Dietary Fiber 4g); Protein 5g.

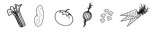

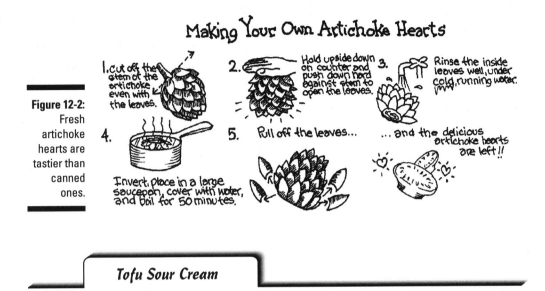

Figure 12-2:
Fresh artichoke hearts are tastier than canned ones.

Tofu Sour Cream

In this recipe, tofu and lemon juice combine to make a dairy-free substitute for sour cream. Use this as the base in all your favorite dip recipes that call for sour cream, or add a dollop — plain or mixed with chopped chives — on a baked potato.

Preparation time: *10 minutes*

Chilling time: *At least 2 hours*

Yield: *12 servings (1½ cups)*

1 10.5-ounce package of silken tofu, any variety of firmness

3 tablespoons vegetable oil

3 tablespoons lemon juice

1 teaspoon clover honey (optional for taste)

1 Combine all the ingredients in a blender or food processor. Blend on high speed until smooth, about 2 to 3 minutes.

2 Transfer the mixture to a glass container, cover, and chill at least 2 hours before serving. Keep in the refrigerator for 5 to 7 days.

Tip: *Store foods with acidic ingredients, such as lemon juice, in nonreactive containers like glass, plastic, or stainless-steel bowls. Aluminum and copper bowls may react with acidic ingredients and cause an off flavor.*

Per serving: *Calories 47 (38 from Fat); Fat 4g (Saturated 0g); Cholesterol 0mg; Sodium 9mg; Carbohydrate 1g (Dietary Fiber 0g); Protein 2g*

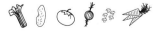

Bean and Cheese Dip

Thick and creamy, this dip is a nutritious comfort food. Serve it hot as an appetizer with your favorite tortilla chips and salsa. Leftovers are good as a sandwich spread. Soy cheese works especially well in this recipe because of its great meltability. Be on the lookout, though, for casein in the ingredient list and avoid brands that contain it if you're allergic to this protein and dairy byproduct. Other styles of nondairy cheese work fine, too. Just be sure to grate them before adding them to the beans to help them melt.

Preparation time: *10 minutes*

Cooking time: *10 minutes*

Yield: *Eight ¼-cup servings*

One 15-ounce can pinto beans, rinsed and drained

½ cup warm water

Half a small white or yellow onion, minced

2 teaspoons minced garlic

¼ cup mild, prepared salsa

6 ounces nondairy cheddar-style cheese, grated

1 Combine the beans and water in a 2-quart saucepan. Cook over medium heat for 2 to 3 minutes, or until the beans are hot.

2 Remove from the heat and mash the beans well with a potato masher or fork. Add the onion and garlic and stir well.

3 Return the mixture to the stovetop and heat on low for 5 minutes, stirring constantly.

4 Stir in the salsa and grated cheese, and heat until the beans are hot and bubbly. Add more water by the tablespoon, if necessary, until the dip reaches the desired consistency.

5 Remove from the heat and serve.

Vary It! *In this recipe, the onions remain crunchy. If you prefer the onions to be cooked, sauté them for a few minutes in a teaspoon of olive oil before adding them to the beans in Step 2. You can substitute black beans in place of the pinto beans and pepper-jack-style nondairy cheese in place of the cheddar-style nondairy cheese.*

Tip: *This bean dip thickens over time. Reheat leftover dip and use it as a filling for tacos and burritos.*

Per serving: *Calories 80 (21 from Fat); Fat 2g (Saturated 0g); Cholesterol 0mg; Sodium 362mg; Carbohydrate 6g (Dietary Fiber 2g); Protein 7g.*

Spreading Some Cheer

Spreads are thick pastes or purées that are smeared onto crackers and breads using a knife or small, flat-bladed spreader. Like dips, they make good appetizers and party foods, and leftovers can be used on toast and as sandwich fillings. This section includes two dairy-free spread recipes.

Maple Nut Spread

This quirky recipe makes a dense, smooth, creamy, not-too-sweet spread similar to cream cheese. This spread works well on a bagel or slice of toast. What better way to start your morning? Or spread it on graham crackers, and you've got a sweet afternoon snack.

Preparation time: *15 minutes*

Cooking time: *40 minutes*

Yield: *8 servings (2 cups)*

⅓ cup raisins or currants	½ teaspoon cinnamon
½ cup very hot water	1 tablespoon tahini
½ pound firm tofu	2 teaspoons pure vanilla extract
¼ cup plain or vanilla soy yogurt	2 teaspoons all-purpose flour
½ cup pure maple syrup	⅓ cup chopped walnuts

1 Preheat the oven to 350 degrees. Lightly grease a 1-quart baking dish or casserole dish.

2 Place the raisins or currants in a small bowl or cup and pour the hot water over them. Set them aside to soak for a few minutes while you work on the next step.

3 Place the tofu, soy yogurt, maple syrup, cinnamon, tahini, vanilla, and flour in a blender or food processor. Blend well, stopping frequently to scrape the sides with a rubber spatula. Turn the ingredients with the spatula if necessary to facilitate thorough blending.

4 Drain the soaked raisins and chop them into small pieces (or give them a whirl in a blender or food processor). Add the raisins and walnuts to the tofu mixture and blend well.

5 Pour the tofu mixture into the prepared baking dish and bake, uncovered, for 40 minutes, or until set. Cool completely before serving. This mixture keeps in the refrigerator for up to 3 days.

Vary It! *For a stronger maple flavor, add ½ teaspoon maple extract in Step 3.*

Per serving: *Calories 143 (46 from Fat); Fat 5g (Saturated 1g); Cholesterol 0mg; Sodium 15mg; Carbohydrate 22g (Dietary Fiber 1g); Protein 4g.*

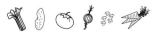

Baked Garlic Spread

This simple but elegant spread will fill your home with the most delicious aroma. It also wins the award for shortest ingredient list. Smear baked garlic on chunks of French or Italian bread. Just reconsider before you kiss someone; keep some breath mints nearby just in case.

Preparation time: 5 minutes

Cooking time: 60 minutes

Yield: 4 servings

1 large bulb of garlic   2 teaspoons olive oil

1 Preheat the oven to 350 degrees. Pull the outer, loose layers of tissue off the garlic bulb, leaving enough so that the cloves remain intact.

2 With a sharp knife, cut off the top of the bulb (about ¼ inch of the top — see Figure 12-3) to expose the tops of the cloves inside. Drizzle the tops of the cloves with the olive oil.

3 Wrap the bulb loosely in aluminum foil, seal the foil completely, and place in the preheated oven.

4 Bake for about 1 hour, or until the cloves are soft. Remove from the oven.

5 Place the garlic bulb on a small serving dish. Lift the softened cloves out of the bulb with a dinner knife and smear them on slices of bread. If the cloves are difficult to remove from bulb, squeeze the bulbs to loosen them first.

Per serving: Calories 33 (21 from Fat); Fat 2g (Saturated 0g); Cholesterol 0mg; Sodium 2mg; Carbohydrate 3g (Dietary Fiber 0g); Protein 1g.

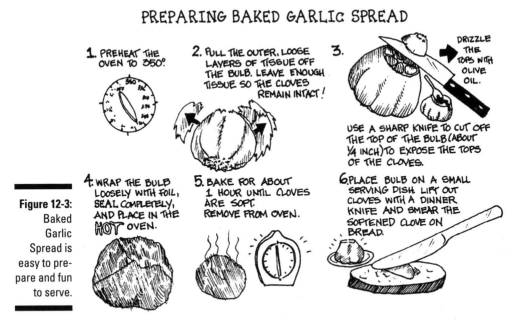

PREPARING BAKED GARLIC SPREAD

1. PREHEAT THE OVEN TO 350°.

2. PULL THE OUTER, LOOSE LAYERS OF TISSUE OFF THE BULB. LEAVE ENOUGH TISSUE SO THE CLOVES REMAIN INTACT!

3. DRIZZLE THE TOPS WITH OLIVE OIL.

USE A SHARP KNIFE TO CUT OFF THE TOP OF THE BULB (ABOUT ¼ INCH) TO EXPOSE THE TOPS OF THE CLOVES.

4. WRAP THE BULB LOOSELY WITH FOIL, SEAL COMPLETELY, AND PLACE IN THE HOT OVEN.

5. BAKE FOR ABOUT 1 HOUR UNTIL CLOVES ARE SOFT. REMOVE FROM OVEN.

6. PLACE BULB ON A SMALL SERVING DISH. LIFT OUT CLOVES WITH A DINNER KNIFE AND SMEAR THE SOFTENED CLOVE ON BREAD.

Figure 12-3: Baked Garlic Spread is easy to prepare and fun to serve.

Sauces for All Seasons

Sauces are liquid or semi-solid toppings added as a complement to a wide range of foods, including meats, casseroles, and other main dishes — even pancakes and desserts. Sauces add color, moisture, and flavor to other foods. Think of them as accessories. You should take full advantage of the power of sauces to elevate the appeal of many of the foods you serve. My three favorite all-purpose dairy-free sauces are

- ✔ Flavorful pesto — usually made with lots of fragrant, fresh basil, Parmesan cheese, nuts, and olive oil

- ✔ Simple marinara sauce, a tomato-based, traditional Italian topping for pasta

- ✔ Alfredo cream sauce — the style you get when you order fettuccine Alfredo at your favorite Italian restaurant

Although all three sauces are perfect for pasta dishes, I use them in other ways, too. For example, I smear French bread rounds with pesto, top them with grated, nondairy Swiss- or mozzarella-style cheese, and toast them in the oven for a quick snack. Marinara sauce is good over a baked potato or on grilled eggplant or *polenta* (cornmeal) cakes. Alfredo cream sauce works well with elbow macaroni for a twist on the usual recipe for macaroni and cheese. You can find many uses for all three of these sauces. Or go crazy and combine all three sauces for the best of all worlds.

Spinach and Basil Pesto Sauce

Pesto usually is made with Parmesan cheese. In this version, *miso,* a savory fermented soy product, and nutritional yeast, both available at natural foods stores, give this sauce its rich flavor. Pesto sauce makes a good dressing for pasta salad; you also can toss it with steamed green beans or mixed vegetables for a change of pace. And spreading it on sandwiches makes lunch less than boring.

Preparation time: *20 minutes*

Yield: *About 1 cup of pesto (which will cover 4 servings of pasta)*

2 cups of loosely packed fresh spinach leaves, stems removed

2 cups of loosely packed fresh basil leaves

½ cup loosely packed fresh parsley

¼ cup toasted pine nuts

3 cloves of garlic, peeled

½ cup extra-virgin olive oil

2 tablespoons water

3 tablespoons white or red miso

3 tablespoons nutritional yeast (optional)

Freshly ground black pepper to taste

1 In a food processor, chop the spinach, basil, parsley, pine nuts, and garlic.

2 Add the olive oil, water, miso, and nutritional yeast (if desired). Continue to process to make a smooth paste. Add black pepper to taste.

Tip: *For a milder garlic flavor, first sauté the garlic in a dry skillet until the papery skin is splotchy brown and the garlic is softened. Next, cool and peel the garlic and then place it in the food processor as noted in the recipe.*

Per serving: *Calories 327 (287 from Fat); Fat 32g (Saturated 4g); Cholesterol 0mg; Sodium 370mg; Carbohydrate 8g (Dietary Fiber 2g); Protein 4g.*

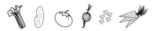

Marinara Sauce

Depending on the season and the amount of time you have, you have two choices with this recipe: fresh or canned tomatoes. In the summertime, nothing is better than home-made marinara sauce made with fresh Italian plum tomatoes. Other times of the year, use canned Italian plum tomatoes — they're still delicious and quicker, too. No matter which way you prepare it, this recipe is great over your favorite pasta.

Preparation time: *15 minutes*

Cooking time: *30 minutes*

Yield: *4 servings (About 2 cups of sauce)*

¼ cup olive oil

1 large white or yellow onion, chopped

3 cloves of garlic, minced

3 pounds of fresh, ripe Italian plum tomatoes, quartered, with seeds removed, or one 28-ounce can of Italian plum tomatoes

Several large basil leaves, shredded

2 teaspoons dried oregano, or a few tablespoons of fresh, chopped

Salt and freshly ground black pepper to taste

1 In a large saucepan, heat 2 tablespoons of the olive oil and add the onions and garlic, cooking over medium heat until the onions are translucent, about 3 minutes.

2 Add the tomatoes. Cook uncovered over medium heat for about 20 minutes, stirring often to prevent sticking. If using fresh tomatoes, press the tomatoes through a strainer and discard the peels and any remaining seeds. Return sauce to pan.

3 Add basil, oregano, salt and pepper, and remaining olive oil. Cook over medium heat for an additional 10 minutes. Serve hot.

Vary It! *Add ½ pound ground turkey or soy burger or sausage crumbles in Step 2. Also consider adding steamed or sautéed veggies (mushrooms, carrots, yellow squash, or whatever you have on hand) to the sauce to add texture, flavor, and nutrition to the sauce.*

Per serving: *Calories 212 (133 from Fat); Fat 15g (Saturated 2g); Cholesterol 0mg; Sodium 178mg; Carbohydrate 21g (Dietary Fiber 5g); Protein 4g.*

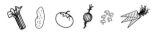

Tofu Alfredo Cream Sauce

In this recipe, the cream and Parmesan cheese used in traditional recipes for Alfredo sauce are replaced by *silken tofu*, a smooth soy product with a custard-like texture, and a soy-based Parmesan cheese-flavored alternative. Walnuts help add the nutty flavor of Parmesan cheese. Despite the substitutions, this recipe can make your pasta Alfredo sing.

Preparation time: *10 minutes*

Yield: *4 servings (about 3 cups)*

One 10.5-ounce package of soft, silken tofu

½ cup plain soymilk

1 tablespoon tahini

1 tablespoon white miso

1 tablespoon lemon juice

¼ teaspoon ground nutmeg

1 cup soy-based or other nondairy Parmesan-style cheese substitute

¼ cup toasted walnuts, finely chopped

Freshly ground black pepper to taste

1 Place all the ingredients in a blender or food processor. Blend until smooth, about 2 minutes.

2 Heat the mixture over medium heat in a small saucepan until hot but not boiling, about 3 minutes. Toss with hot pasta and serve immediately.

Per serving: Calories 232 (96 from Fat); Fat 11g (Saturated 1g); Cholesterol 0mg; Sodium 136mg; Carbohydrate 16g (Dietary Fiber 9g); Protein 23g.

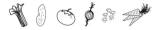

Making Dairy-Free Dressings

The good news for you — the dear reader who wants to go dairy-free — is that some of the best salad dressings are made with nothing more than vegetable or extra-virgin olive oil, vinegar, herbs, and spices. Using your imagination and adding bits of fresh fruit or fruit juices, ground nuts and seeds, and other wholesome ingredients can make delicious variations.

If you're more into creamy dressings, you're still in luck. You can make creamy, nondairy salad dressings just by thinning plain soy yogurt with a bit of fruit juice or nondairy milk and adding your choice of fresh herbs.

The recipes I provide in this section are dairy-free versions of two of the most popular salad dressings — creamy Italian and Ranch. Experiment with your favorite ingredients and create other unique dressings of your own.

Creamy Italian Dressing

Not only is this dressing good on a green salad, it also works well on pasta salad and as an all-purpose dressing for pita pocket sandwiches filled with shredded vegetables, greens, and grated nondairy cheese. Creamy and very tasty, this is a good, low-cost, and dairy-free replacement for store-bought dressing.

Preparation time: *5 minutes*

Chilling time: *At least 2 hours*

Yield: *10 servings (about 1¼ cups)*

1 cup soy or regular mayonnaise

3 tablespoons plain nondairy milk

1 tablespoon red wine vinegar

2 cloves of garlic, minced

½ teaspoon sugar

¼ teaspoon white pepper

1 teaspoon dried basil leaves or a few fresh leaves, chopped

1 teaspoon dried oregano or a couple of fresh sprigs, chopped

1 Place all the ingredients in a blender or food processor. Blend until smooth, about 2 minutes.

2 Chill for at least 2 hours before serving. Keep in the refrigerator for five to seven days.

Vary It! *Add 3 tablespoons more vinegar if you like your dressing a little thinner and tarter.*

Per serving: *Calories 163 (159 from Fat); Fat 18g (Saturated 3g); Cholesterol 13mg; Sodium 126mg; Carbohydrate 1g (Dietary Fiber 0g); Protein 1g.*

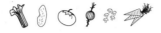

Green Goodness Ranch Dressing

Who says Ranch dressing has to be white? For readers who are old enough to remember, this dressing also is known as Green Goddess. The origins of this dressing are uncertain, but it was a popular store-bought dressing in the early 1970s before Ranch dressing came onto the scene. The original contained sour cream and was distinctive for its green hue. This version replaces sour cream with a nondairy alternative. The dressing also makes a good dip for vegetables.

Preparation time: *5 minutes*

Chilling time: *At least 2 hours*

Yield: *10 servings (1¼ cups)*

½ cup plain nondairy sour cream

½ cup soy or regular mayonnaise

3 tablespoons tahini

1 tablespoon honey

2 tablespoons fresh parsley, chopped

1 green onion, chopped

¼ teaspoon white pepper

2 cloves of garlic, minced

1 teaspoon dried chives, or a few fresh leaves, chopped

1 teaspoon dried tarragon, or a couple of sprigs, chopped

1 Place all the ingredients in a blender or food processor. Blend until smooth, about 2 minutes.

2 Chill for at least 2 hours before serving.

Per serving: Calories 135 (119 from Fat); Fat 13g (Saturated 2g); Cholesterol 7mg; Sodium 113mg; Carbohydrate 4g (Dietary Fiber 0g); Protein 1g.

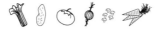

Chapter 13

Breads, Pizza, and Munchies

In This Chapter

▶ Baking homemade breads without dairy

▶ Making tasty nondairy pizza

▶ Assembling traditional snacks the dairy-free way

Most of your favorite recipes for baked goods and snacks probably include dairy products in some form. I have some good news for you: You don't have to give up bread, pizza, and other snacks just because you want to eliminate dairy from your diet.

You can make all three with dairy-free ingredients. Breads often call for milk or buttermilk, but they're easily replaced with nondairy alternatives. As for pizza, you've probably never had it made without cheese. Get ready to be pleasantly surprised. When pizza is topped with rich tomato sauce and flavorful toppings, the absence of cheese is likely to go unnoticed. But, if you can't go without cheese, don't worry. I also include a recipe for a Greek-style pizza that is topped with nondairy mozzarella. Snacks and appetizers, too, often incorporate nondairy cheese as a key ingredient.

The recipes I include in this chapter are only a sample of the range of breads, pizzas, and snacks you can make without adding an ounce of dairy. They're simply a good demonstration of the versatility of the dairy substitutes on the market as well as an illustration of the appeal of some foods that include no dairy ingredients or substitutes at all.

Falling in Love with Dairy-Free Breads

Bread has a special place in many people's hearts, and it can be used in so many ways. Freshly baked bread fills your home with an aroma so good that real estate agents often recommend it as a strategy for making buyers fall in love your home. Bread also adds variety and rounds out meals. A warm roll, a chunk of crusty bread, or a warm slice of toast can be all you need to make a meal out of a bowl of soup or a salad.

I include four examples of easy-to-make breads in this section. One is made with no dairy or dairy substitutes at all, and the others incorporate a range of nondairy alternatives. No need for a new cookbook just because you're going dairy-free — just use these examples to help guide you in adapting your other favorite bread recipes.

Whole-wheat and white pita pocket bread and flour tortillas often are made without dairy ingredients (always read the ingredient list to make sure, though). Buy them ready-made and use them as alternatives to loaf bread for sandwiches.

Cheddar Cheese Bread

This rich-tasting bread contains no saturated fat because it's made with nondairy cheese instead of traditional cheddar cheese. Serve a chunk of this bread with a bowl of chili or black bean soup, or toast a couple slices to make sandwiches filled with fresh spinach leaves, tomato slices, chopped black olives, and a splash of vinaigrette dressing.

Preparation time: *30 minutes, plus rising time of at least 1 hour*

Cooking time: *60 minutes*

Yield: *2 loaves (12 slices per loaf)*

6 cups all-purpose flour	*1 package (¼ ounce) active dry yeast*
1½ teaspoons salt	*1¾ cups lukewarm water*
1 tablespoon granulated sugar	*¾ cup cheddar-style nondairy cheese*
1 tablespoon olive oil	*1 tablespoon black pepper*

1 Stir together the flour, salt, sugar, and olive oil in a medium mixing bowl.

2 Combine the yeast and water in a small cup and stir until the yeast is dissolved. Pour the yeast mixture into the flour mixture and mix thoroughly in an electric stand mixer with a dough hook, in a food processor, or with your hands.

3 Remove the dough from the bowl, turn onto a floured surface, and knead for 10 minutes by hand or with a machine. (Figure 13-1 shows the proper technique for kneading bread dough with your hands.) If the dough is too dry, you can drizzle up to ⅓ cup additional water to make the dough stick together.

4 Oil a large bowl with olive oil. Place the dough ball in the bowl, and then turn it over once so that you lightly coat the top of the dough ball with oil. Cover the dough with a towel or waxed paper, and let it rise in a warm place (under a sunny window or on top of a warm stove, for example) until it has doubled in size, about 1 hour.

5 On a floured surface (or in the bowl of a mixer or food processor), combine the cheese and black pepper and then knead the dough into the cheese mixture. Continue kneading for 6 or 7 minutes, or until the cheese and pepper are well incorporated into the dough.

6 Divide the dough into 2 balls. Place each ball into an oiled 9-x-5-x-3-inch loaf pan. Cover the loaf pans and let the dough rise for 30 minutes to 1 hour, or until it reaches to just above the top of the loaf pan. Preheat the oven to 350 degrees.

7 Bake the loaves for 60 minutes, or until the bread is browned on top and sounds hollow when thumped with your knuckles. Remove from the oven, let cool, and serve.

Vary It! Add 2 teaspoons chopped dill or another favorite herb in Step 6.

Per serving: Calories 130 (11 from Fat); Fat 1g (Saturated 0g); Cholesterol 0mg; Sodium 188mg; Carbohydrate 25g (Dietary Fiber 1g); Protein 4g.

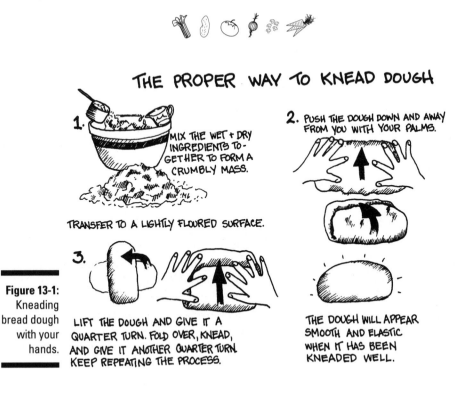

THE PROPER WAY TO KNEAD DOUGH

1. MIX THE WET + DRY INGREDIENTS TOGETHER TO FORM A CRUMBLY MASS.

TRANSFER TO A LIGHTLY FLOURED SURFACE.

2. PUSH THE DOUGH DOWN AND AWAY FROM YOU WITH YOUR PALMS.

3. LIFT THE DOUGH AND GIVE IT A QUARTER TURN. FOLD OVER, KNEAD, AND GIVE IT ANOTHER QUARTER TURN. KEEP REPEATING THE PROCESS.

THE DOUGH WILL APPEAR SMOOTH AND ELASTIC WHEN IT HAS BEEN KNEADED WELL.

Figure 13-1: Kneading bread dough with your hands.

Banana Bread

Everybody loves banana bread. This quick bread is moist and sweet with a mild banana flavor. In this recipe, oil is substituted for butter, making the bread dairy-free. Half of the flour used is whole wheat, boosting the nutritional value of the recipe by adding dietary fiber and trace minerals. For a change of pace, try using banana bread to make the Easy French Toast recipe in Chapter 9. And try freezing slices of this bread individually so you'll always have a tasty breakfast within reach!

Preparation time: *15 minutes*

Cooking time: *60 to 70 minutes*

Yield: *1 loaf (12 slices)*

½ cup vegetable oil

1 cup sugar

2 eggs (or equivalent amount of cholesterol-free egg replacer)

2 medium ripe bananas, mashed

1½ cups all-purpose flour

½ cup whole-wheat flour

1 teaspoon baking powder

½ teaspoon baking soda

½ teaspoon salt

½ cup chopped walnuts or pecans (optional)

1 Preheat the oven to 350 degrees. In a medium bowl, whisk together the oil, sugar, and eggs. Add the bananas and blend well with an electric mixer.

2 In a separate bowl, combine the flour, baking powder, baking soda, and salt. Add this mixture to the banana mixture gradually, beating well between additions. Stir the nuts into the finished batter (if desired).

3 Pour the batter into an oiled 9-x-5-x-3-inch loaf pan and bake for 60 to 70 minutes, or until the bread is golden brown. Cool on a wire rack in the pan. When the loaf is cool enough to handle, remove from the pan and serve.

Vary It! *Add 6 ounces of carob chips or dairy-free chocolate chips to the finished batter in Step 2.*

Per serving: *Calories 252 (94 from Fat); Fat 10g (Saturated 1g); Cholesterol 35mg; Sodium 192mg; Carbohydrate 37g (Dietary Fiber 2g); Protein 4g.*

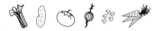

Country Cornbread

Soy yogurt helps to moisten this bread while keeping it dairy-free. Bits of corn add texture. The flavor is similar to that of cornbread made with dairy. The bread crumbles easily and melts in your mouth. Serve it with Cream of Tomato Soup (see Chapter 10) or a bowl of your favorite chili.

Preparation time: *5 minutes*

Cooking time: *30 minutes*

Yield: *4 servings*

2 tablespoons olive oil plus 1 tablespoon extra to oil the casserole dish (or use vegetable oil spray)

¾ cup cornmeal

⅓ cup canned corn, drained

2 egg whites (or equivalent amount of cholesterol-free egg replacer)

1½ cups plain soy yogurt

½ teaspoon baking soda

½ teaspoon salt

½ cup chopped white or yellow onion

¼ teaspoon black pepper

1 Preheat the oven to 425 degrees. Oil a 1-quart casserole dish or oven-safe cast-iron skillet.

2 Combine all the ingredients in a medium-sized bowl and stir until completely mixed.

3 Pour the batter into the prepared dish or skillet and bake for 30 minutes, or until set. (To test for doneness, stick a toothpick into the bread. If it comes out clean, the bread is done.) Be careful not to overbake.

Vary It! *Add ¼ cup sliced jalapeño peppers for an extra kick or chopped sun-dried tomatoes to Step 2 for a savory flavor.*

Per serving: Calories 257 (105 from Fat); Fat 12g (Saturated 2g); Cholesterol 0mg; Sodium 532mg; Carbohydrate 33g (Dietary Fiber 3g); Protein 6g.

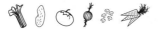

Multigrain Crescent Rolls

I love the soft, slightly chewy texture of these rolls. They keep for two or three days in an airtight bag, and they freeze well, too. You can use them in a wide variety of ways: Dollop a little jam on one in the morning for breakfast, nibble on one for an afternoon snack, or use one to dab your leftover dressing with a salad. In this recipe, soymilk replaces cow's milk to make these rolls dairy-free.

Preparation time: *15 minutes, plus 2½ hours for the dough to rise*

Cooking time: *15 minutes*

Yield: *32 rolls*

1 package (¼ ounce) active dry yeast

¼ cup lukewarm water

¾ cup soymilk

2 tablespoons sugar

2 tablespoons honey

1 teaspoon salt

2 egg whites (or equivalent amount of cholesterol-free egg replacer)

¼ cup vegetable oil, plus extra for oiling the dough

1½ cups whole-wheat flour

2 cups all-purpose flour

Olive oil (for oiling bowl)

1 In a large mixing bowl, dissolve the yeast completely in the water. Set aside. Warm the soymilk in a saucepan over low heat for 3 or 4 minutes, or until lukewarm to the touch.

2 Add the warmed soymilk, sugar, honey, salt, egg whites, ¼ cup oil, and whole-wheat flour to the yeast. Stir until all the ingredients are well combined and the dough is smooth. Add the all-purpose flour and mix until the dough forms a ball. If the dough is too sticky to handle, add several more tablespoons of all-purpose flour as necessary. (If you don't want to mix by hand, a stand mixer with a paddle attachment works well.)

3 Place the dough on a floured surface and knead for several minutes until it's smooth and elastic. (See Figure 13-1 earlier in the chapter for instructions on how to knead dough by hand.)

4 Oil a large bowl with olive oil. Place the dough ball in the bowl, and then turn it over once so you lightly coat the top of the dough ball with oil. Cover the bowl with a towel or waxed paper, and let the dough rise in a warm place (under a sunny window or on top of a warm stove, for example) until doubled in size, about 2 hours. Punch down the dough ball with your fist, and then divide the ball into 2 pieces.

5 Place the dough balls, one at a time, on a floured surface. Roll each piece of dough into a circle approximately 12 inches in diameter. Lightly brush each circle with vegetable oil. With a sharp knife, cut the circle in half, and then in quarters, continuing until you have 16 wedges of dough. (See Figure 13-2.)

6 Preheat the oven to 350 degrees. Beginning at the wide end of each wedge, roll the dough into a crescent shape, ending by pressing the tip onto the roll. Set each roll on a lightly oiled baking sheet and bend the ends slightly to give the roll a crescent shape.

7 Cover and let the rolls rise for about 30 minutes before baking. Bake the rolls for 15 minutes, or until they're lightly browned. Be careful not to overbake.

Per serving: Calories 75 (20 from Fat); Fat 2g (Saturated 0g); Cholesterol 0mg; Sodium 77mg; Carbohydrate 12g (Dietary Fiber 1g); Protein 2g.

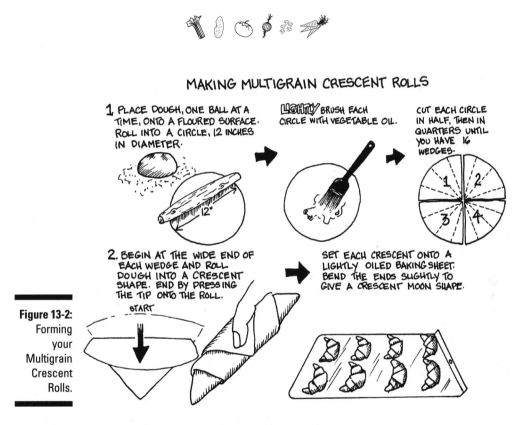

MAKING MULTIGRAIN CRESCENT ROLLS

1. PLACE DOUGH, ONE BALL AT A TIME, ONTO A FLOURED SURFACE. ROLL INTO A CIRCLE, 12 INCHES IN DIAMETER.

LIGHTLY BRUSH EACH CIRCLE WITH VEGETABLE OIL.

CUT EACH CIRCLE IN HALF, THEN IN QUARTERS UNTIL YOU HAVE 16 WEDGES.

2. BEGIN AT THE WIDE END OF EACH WEDGE AND ROLL DOUGH INTO A CRESCENT SHAPE. END BY PRESSING THE TIP ONTO THE ROLL.

START

SET EACH CRESCENT ONTO A LIGHTLY OILED BAKING SHEET. BEND THE ENDS SLIGHTLY TO GIVE A CRESCENT MOON SHAPE.

Figure 13-2: Forming your Multigrain Crescent Rolls.

Kneading Some Pizza

Most people love to sink their teeth into a hot pizza pie. If you're a fan of pizzas, you'll love these versions, too. However, if you've not been a fan of pizza because you're lactose intolerant and the cheesy pies give your stomach fits, the cramping can now end. These two nondairy recipes begin with a simple, homemade pizza crust that's easy to make.

If you have young children, pizza is a good recipe to get them involved in making. Let kids help to knead the dough and arrange the toppings. They'll enjoy eating a meal they had a hand in making.

If you miss the flavor of cheese on your pizza, try adding a bit of soy-based Parmesan cheese. Sprinkle a little over the top of the pizza. *Nutritional yeast,* available at natural foods stores, is a savory, flaked yeast product that resembles Parmesan cheese in flavor. It's another dairy-free option that makes a good condiment for pizza.

Cheeseless Pizza

This recipe is made just like any other pizza minus the cheese. The sauce and toppings add so much color and flavor that your family or friends may not even notice the cheese is missing. This recipe makes two large pizzas.

Preparation time: *About 90 minutes (including time for the dough to rise)*

Cooking time: *30 minutes*

Yield: *2 large pizzas (about 8 slices per pizza)*

Pizza Dough

1½ teaspoons active dry yeast

1¾ cup warm water (110 degrees)

1 tablespoon honey or sugar

1 teaspoon olive oil, plus extra for oiling the bowl and dough

½ teaspoon salt

2 cups whole-wheat flour

2 cups all-purpose flour

1 In a large mixing bowl, dissolve the yeast in the warm water and add the honey or sugar. Add the teaspoon of oil and the salt and stir.

2 Gradually add the flour, alternating between whole-wheat and white. Mix well after each addition using a wooden spoon or your hands to make a soft dough.

3 Turn out the dough onto a floured board and knead for 5 minutes, adding more flour if necessary. (See Figure 13-1 earlier in the chapter to see how to properly knead dough by hand.)

4 Lightly oil the sides of the mixing bowl. Put the dough back into the bowl, turn the dough over once to coat with oil, cover with a towel or waxed paper, and then let it set in a warm place (under a sunny window or on top of a warm stove, for example) for about 60 minutes.

5 Divide the dough in half. Reserve one half for later, if desired (store in the refrigerator or freezer).

Assembling the Pizza

1 cup of chopped vegetables, including broccoli, mushrooms, green or red bell peppers, onions, black olives, pineapple chunks, and so on

1 recipe pizza dough (see the preceding recipe)

1 cup prepared pizza sauce (more or less to suit your taste)

Soy Parmesan cheese for garnish, if desired

1 Preheat the oven to 375 degrees and wash and chop the vegetables. Set aside.

2 Spread the pizza dough (see preceding recipe) on an oiled, 14-inch pizza pan. You can roll the dough out first on a floured surface or simply press the ball of dough onto the pizza pan and distribute it evenly using your hands.

3 Spoon on the pizza sauce and spread it to within ½ inch of the edge of the dough. Add the vegetables.

4 Place the pizza in the oven and bake for 30 minutes, or until the crust begins to brown lightly. Be careful not to overbake.

5 Remove the pizza from the oven, and let it sit for 5 minutes. Cut the pizza into slices and serve. Sprinkle some nondairy Parmesan cheese on the pizza slices, if desired.

Vary It! *Add 8 ounces diced chicken or soy-based chicken or veggie pepperoni slices in Step 3.*

Tip: *When you make pizza from scratch, make extra dough and freeze it for later. That way, you'll have it ready for a day when you need to make dinner in a hurry. Thaw the dough completely in the refrigerator or on the kitchen counter before using. Pizza dough keeps in the freezer for up to three months.*

Per slice: Calories 160 (25 from Fat); Fat 3g (Saturated 0g); Cholesterol 0mg; Sodium 459mg; Carbohydrate 29g (Dietary Fiber 4g); Protein 5g.

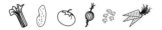

Greek Pizza

This pizza recipe is more traditional but uses a mozzarella-style cheese substitute in lieu of dairy cheese. Greek pizza is so named because the toppings — spinach, red onions, and Kalamata olives — are so popular in many Greek dishes. You'll love them on this pizza, too!

Preparation time: *About 90 minutes (including time for the dough to rise)*

Cooking time: *30 minutes*

Yield: *2 large pizzas (about 8 slices per pizza)*

Pizza Dough

1½ teaspoons active dry yeast

1¾ cup warm water (110 degrees)

1 teaspoon olive oil, plus extra for oiling the bowl and dough

1 tablespoon honey or sugar

½ teaspoon salt

2 cups whole-wheat flour

2 cups all-purpose flour

1 In a large mixing bowl, dissolve the yeast in the warm water and add the honey or sugar. Add the teaspoon of oil and the salt and stir.

2 Gradually add the flour, alternating between whole-wheat and white. Mix well after each addition using a wooden spoon or your hands to make a soft dough.

3 Turn out the dough onto a floured board and knead for 5 minutes, adding more flour if necessary. (See Figure 13-1 earlier in the chapter to see how to properly knead dough by hand.)

4 Lightly oil the sides of the mixing bowl. Put the dough back into the bowl, turn the dough over once to coat with oil, cover with a towel or waxed paper, and then let set in a warm place (under a sunny window or on top of a warm stove, for example) for about 60 minutes.

5 Divide the dough in half. Reserve one half for later, if desired (store in the refrigerator or freezer).

Assembling the Pizza

4 cups baby spinach leaves

3 to 4 large Roma tomatoes, sliced

Half of a red onion, thinly sliced

½ cup sliced Kalamata or black olives

1 recipe pizza dough (see preceding recipe)

1 cup prepared pizza sauce (more or less to suit your taste)

2 cups shredded mozzarella-style nondairy cheese

1 Preheat the oven to 375 degrees and wash and slice the vegetables. Set aside.

2 Spread the prepared dough (see preceding recipe) on a 14-inch pizza pan. You can roll the dough out first on a floured surface or simply press the ball of dough onto the pizza pan and distribute it evenly using your hands.

3 Spoon on the pizza sauce and spread it to within ½ inch of the edge of the dough. Add the vegetable toppings.

4 Place the pizza in the oven and bake for 20 minutes, or until the crust begins to brown lightly. Be careful not to overbake.

5 Remove the pizza from the oven and then sprinkle the shredded mozzarella-style non-dairy cheese evenly over the pizza. Place the pizza back into the oven for another 10 minutes.

6 Remove the pizza from the oven and let it sit for 5 minutes. Cut into slices and serve.

Vary It! *Some natural foods stores carry a soy-based substitute for feta cheese, a goat milk cheese popular in Greek and Middle Eastern cooking. Try it in Step 4 in lieu of mozzarella-style cheese.*

Per slice: Calories 227 (61 from Fat); Fat 7g (Saturated 0g); Cholesterol 0mg; Sodium 408mg; Carbohydrate 30g (Dietary Fiber 4g); Protein 12g.

Satisfying Cravings at Snack Time

Who doesn't like to munch on snacks while watching movies or TV? Let's face it: Snacks are a (fun) fact of life! Unfortunately for dairy-free eaters, cheese figures prominently in many favorite snack foods. But don't worry. You don't need to avoid your favorite cheesy snacks. Just substitute non-dairy cheeses.

The two examples in this section — cheesy nachos and hot, flavorful bruschetta — are versatile favorites. Serve either as a quick snack or as an appetizer. If you increase the portion size and add a green salad, both of these make a delicious lunch or dinner.

Mucho Nachos

These nachos are made with nondairy cheese substitute and nondairy sour cream topping. Your guests won't notice the difference between this version and one made with dairy-based toppings — especially when you top them with all the other traditional toppings, including jalapeños, guacamole, and salsa. Soy cheese works well in this recipe because of its superior melting quality, but read ingredient labels because some brands contain the milk protein casein.

Preparation time: *15 minutes*

Cooking time: *About 10 minutes*

Yield: *6 heaping servings*

One 22-ounce bag of tortilla chips

Two 15-ounce cans refried black or pinto beans

6 ounces cheddar-style nondairy cheese, grated

1 cup prepared salsa

½ cup sliced black olives

2 jalapeño peppers, sliced (optional)

2 cups chopped Romaine lettuce

1 large tomato, cored, seeded, and chopped

¼ cup nondairy sour cream

½ cup prepared nondairy guacamole (optional)

Additional salsa as desired

1 Preheat the oven to 375 degrees. Spread the chips evenly on an oiled pizza pan or a baking sheet.

2 In a medium saucepan, warm the refried beans over medium heat, stirring to prevent sticking, about 5 minutes. Add tablespoons of water, as needed, to thin the beans to a creamy consistency.

3 Spoon the beans over the chips, and then sprinkle cheese evenly over the chips and beans. Spoon salsa evenly over the chips, beans, and cheese. Top with black olives and jalapeño peppers (if desired).

4 Place the pan into the oven and bake until cheese is melted and lightly browned, about 10 minutes.

5 Remove the nachos from the oven. Top with chopped lettuce, tomato, nondairy sour cream, and guacamole (if desired). Serve with extra salsa.

Vary It! *Add a layer of 8 ounces cooked, ground turkey or soy burger crumbles after the beans in Step 3.*

Per serving: Calories 769 (307 from Fat); Fat 34g (Saturated 3g); Cholesterol 0mg; Sodium 1,351mg; Carbohydrate 96g (Dietary Fiber 15g); Protein 24g.

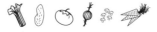

Bruschetta

Bruschetta is an Italian appetizer made with sliced rounds of bread that are brushed with olive oil and toasted in the oven. A variety of toppings are added. Fresh, seasonal tomatoes and basil make this version a perfect summertime treat. Leftovers — in the unlikely event that you have any — are good reheated in the oven. I prefer soy cheese here for its melting quality, but you can use other nondairy varieties as well. (If you do use soy cheese, read the ingredient label to make sure it doesn't contain casein, in case you're sensitive to the milk protein.)

Preparation time: *About 15 minutes*

Cooking time: *About 12 minutes*

Yield: *6 servings*

One French baguette, approximately 18 inches in length

2 tablespoons olive oil, plus extra for brushing over bread rounds

4 medium tomatoes, cored, seeded, and diced (refer to Figure 13-3)

1 cup fresh basil leaves, chopped

6 ounces mozzarella-style soy cheese, grated

3 cloves of garlic, minced

¼ cup balsamic vinegar

1 Preheat the oven to 375 degrees. Slice the baguette crosswise into ¾-inch rounds (a total of 24 rounds). Place rounds on an oiled baking sheet and brush the tops with olive oil.

2 Place the bread into the oven and bake until it's toasted and slightly browned, about 8 minutes. Remove from oven and set aside.

3 Place the tomatoes, basil, soy cheese, garlic, 2 tablespoons olive oil, and vinegar into a medium bowl. Toss to mix well.

4 Distribute tomato mixture evenly on the bread rounds, patting it down slightly to help it stay in place.

5 Place bruschetta back into the oven and heat for about 4 minutes to allow cheese to melt a little. Remove from the oven and serve.

Vary It! *For those who prefer a cheeseless option, leave out the soy cheese in Step 3.*

Per serving: *Calories 255 (117 from Fat); Fat 13g (Saturated 2g); Cholesterol 0mg; Sodium 564mg; Carbohydrate 28g (Dietary Fiber 3g); Protein 9g.*

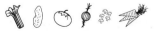

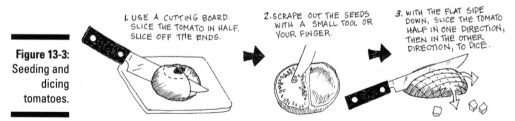

HOW TO SEED AND DICE TOMATOES

Figure 13-3:
Seeding and
dicing
tomatoes.

1. USE A CUTTING BOARD. SLICE THE TOMATO IN HALF. SLICE OFF THE ENDS.

2. SCRAPE OUT THE SEEDS WITH A SMALL TOOL OR YOUR FINGER.

3. WITH THE FLAT SIDE DOWN, SLICE THE TOMATO HALF IN ONE DIRECTION, THEN IN THE OTHER DIRECTION, TO DICE.

Chapter 14

Dishing Up Dairy-Free Desserts

Dessert is one of life's simple pleasures. Giving up dairy doesn't have to mean giving up dessert, though. However, it does increase the likelihood that you'll want to prepare more desserts from scratch at home so you can control the ingredients. That's because so many traditional sweet treats contain milk, cream, sour cream, soft cheeses, and other dairy ingredients. Fortunately, desserts that contain dairy are easy to recreate as dairy-free delights. In this chapter, I show you how.

This chapter has a plethora of dessert options, including smoothies, pudding, pie, cake, and even dairy-free ice cream. Try these recipes for yourself; you can then experiment and create original recipes of your own. My hope is that this chapter gives you the confidence — and inspiration — to tackle any recipe makeover with skill and enthusiasm.

Sipping on Smoothies

Smoothies are the modern adaptation of the old-fashioned milkshake. Although shakes and malts usually are made with ice cream, smoothies typically are made with a wider range of ingredients, including milk, yogurt, fruit, vegetables, crushed ice, frozen yogurt, and other ingredients. Most smoothies also are sweetened with a little maple syrup, honey, or another sweetener. Some have wheat germ, green tea, herbal supplements, and other nutritional supplements added. When you make them with wholesome ingredients, such as nondairy milks and frozen fruit, they can be nutritious snacks.

As blended beverages, smoothies are cold and refreshing and lend themselves to lots of variations. Experiment with different combinations of ingredients. Throw in a frozen banana or a few handfuls of frozen, mixed berries. Use up the last few drops of orange juice or almond milk in the refrigerator.

Ice cubes, crushed in blending, improve the mouth feel or texture of smoothies, making them frostier. For a thicker smoothie, add more ice cubes or frozen fruit until you reach the desired consistency. For a thinner smoothie, add more juice or nondairy milk.

Very Cranberry Smoothie

Sweet strawberries and blueberries complement the tart cranberry flavor and add color to this delicious dessert drink. Use fresh, locally grown fruit for the best flavor. What better treat can there be after a Saturday morning trip to the farmers' market?

Preparation time: *4 minutes*

Yield: *Two 12-ounce servings*

1 cup pure cranberry juice

1½ cups nondairy vanilla frozen ice cream (let it soften a little before you use it so it's easier to measure)

1 cup fresh or frozen strawberries

½ cup fresh or frozen blueberries

2 tablespoons pure maple syrup (or honey)

5 or 6 ice cubes

A few fresh mint leaves

1 Place all the ingredients except the mint leaves in a blender and blend on high speed for about 1 minute, or until smooth, stopping every 15 seconds to scrape the sides of the blender with a spatula and to push the solid ingredients down to the bottom of the blender. Thin the mixture as needed with a little more cranberry juice until it reaches the desired consistency.

2 Pour the blended mixture into two tall, 16-ounce tumblers, garnish with mint leaves, and serve immediately with iced tea spoons and straws.

Tip: Single readers can reserve half the smoothie in the refrigerator for several hours. It won't be as frosty if enjoyed later, but it will still taste good.

Per serving: *Calories 455 (from Fat 154); Fat 17g (Saturated 3g); Cholesterol 0mg; Sodium 322mg; Carbohydrate 73g (Dietary Fiber 3g); Protein 4g.*

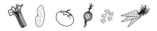

Strawberry Kiwi Smoothie

This smoothie provides a blast of vitamin C as it cools and refreshes. Let the pretty rose color show through by serving it in a tall, clear glass. Use fresh, locally grown berries in season for the best flavor.

Preparation time: *3 minutes*

Yield: *Two 12-ounce servings*

1 cup orange juice

1½ cups nondairy vanilla ice cream

1 cup fresh or frozen strawberries

3 fresh kiwi, peeled and sliced

1 teaspoon pure vanilla extract

2 tablespoons pure maple syrup (or honey)

5 or 6 ice cubes

1 Place all the ingredients in a blender and blend on high speed for about 1 minute, or until smooth, stopping every 15 seconds to scrape the sides of the blender with a spatula and to push the solid ingredients down to the bottom of the blender. Thin the mixture as needed with a little more orange juice until it reaches the desired consistency.

2 Pour into two tall, 16-ounce tumblers and serve immediately with iced tea spoons and straws.

Tip: *Single readers can reserve half the smoothie in the refrigerator for several hours. It won't be as frosty enjoyed later, but it will still taste good.*

Per serving: *Calories 498 (from Fat 161); Fat 18g (Saturated 3g); Cholesterol 0mg; Sodium 319mg; Carbohydrate 80g (Dietary Fiber 5g); Protein 6g.*

Putting Together Perfect Puddings

Puddings are some of the easiest recipes to convert to dairy-free status. Traditional recipes call for cow's milk, but any of the nondairy alternatives work well as substitutes. As I explain in Chapter 8, you can use nondairy milks in exactly the same proportions as cow's milk when you make pudding from scratch. So if your favorite pudding recipe calls for 2 cups of cow's milk, simply substitute 2 cups of nondairy milk — soymilk, almond milk, or rice milk — instead.

The added bonus of making your own nondairy pudding is that by swapping nondairy milk for cow's milk, you reduce the saturated fat content of the pudding without sacrificing flavor or texture. What's not to like about that?

When you make pudding, both vanilla and plain milks work well in the recipes. Use whichever you have on hand or whichever you prefer.

Grandma's Tapioca Pudding

As a child, my mother made heaping, family-sized bowls of homemade tapioca pudding. I don't recall these extra-large batches lasting more than a day. So, of course, I was inspired to create a nondairy version. Soaking the tapioca before cooking gives it time to absorb some of the nondairy milk and helps prevent the scorching that sometimes happens when tapioca beads settle on the bottom of the pan. In the summertime, serve tapioca with fresh strawberries, blueberries, or raspberries.

Preparation time: *5 minutes*

Cooking time: *10 minutes*

Cooling time: *20 minutes*

Yield: *4 servings (about ⅔ cups each)*

½ cup sugar

3 tablespoons quick-cooking tapioca

2¾ cup plain or vanilla soymilk
(or your choice of nondairy milk)

1 egg (or equivalent amount of cholesterol-free egg replacer)

½ teaspoon pure almond extract (optional)

1 In a medium saucepan, combine the sugar, tapioca, soymilk, and egg. Stir and then let soak for 5 minutes.

2 Cook over medium heat, stirring constantly, until the mixture comes to a full boil (about 10 minutes). Remove from the heat.

3 Stir in the almond extract (if desired). Let the tapioca cool for 20 minutes, and then stir again.

4 Spoon the pudding into 6 serving cups or 1 serving bowl. Serve warm or chilled.

Per serving: Calories 214 (from Fat 33); Fat 4g (Saturated 0g); Cholesterol 53mg; Sodium 81mg; Carbohydrate 40g (Dietary Fiber 0g); Protein 6g.

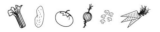

Creamy Rice Pudding
with Cardamom and Raisins

This pudding thickens in the pan as the rice absorbs the liquid in the recipe. The result is a rich, creamy pudding that's simple to make and requires minimal supervision time at the stove — a big plus. The addition of golden raisins and cardamom are a delicious twist on an old favorite.

Preparation time: *5 minutes*

Cooking time: *50 minutes*

Chilling time (optional): *2 hours*

Yield: *6 servings*

3 cups vanilla soymilk (or your choice of nondairy milk)

½ cup long-grain white rice

½ cup golden raisins

¼ teaspoon salt

1 tablespoon nondairy, trans-fat-free margarine

¼ cup sugar

½ teaspoon ground cardamom

1 teaspoon pure vanilla extract

Ground cardamom for garnish (optional)

1 In a medium saucepan, bring the soymilk to a boil over high heat, stirring constantly (about 5 minutes).

2 Add the rice, raisins, salt, margarine, sugar, cardamom, and vanilla. Stir to combine. Reduce the heat to low.

3 Cook, covered, for about 45 minutes, or until all the liquid has been absorbed. Lift the lid and stir every 15 minutes, covering again tightly each time you remove the lid.

4 After all the liquid has been absorbed, remove the pudding from the heat. Cool until only warm. Serve immediately or place in the refrigerator to chill for 2 hours. Top with a sprinkling of ground cardamom, if desired. Pudding can be stored in the refrigerator for a week (but it will be gone before then!).

Vary It! *Substitute chopped dates for raisins. Add ⅓ cup chopped almonds in Step 2. For a richer pudding, try using soy creamer in place of the soymilk.*

Per serving: *Calories 206 (from Fat 34); Fat 4g (Saturated 1g); Cholesterol 0mg; Sodium 168mg; Carbohydrate 37g (Dietary Fiber 1g); Protein 5g.*

Favorite Chocolate Pudding

Chocolate pudding is a classic comfort food. Enjoy this one — dairy-free! Unsweetened cocoa powder gives this pudding a mild chocolate flavor. Pudding lovers may want to double this recipe.

Preparation time: *5 minutes*

Cooking time: *15 minutes*

Chilling time: *2 hours*

Yield: *4 servings*

½ cup sugar

2 tablespoons cornstarch

⅓ cup unsweetened cocoa powder

¼ teaspoon salt

2 cups vanilla or plain soymilk
(or your choice of nondairy milk)

2 tablespoons nondairy, trans-fat-free margarine

2 teaspoons vanilla

1 Combine the sugar, cornstarch, cocoa, and salt in a medium saucepan. Add the milk, stirring to dissolve the sugar mixture.

2 Cook over medium heat, stirring constantly, until the mixture thickens and comes to a full boil (about 10 minutes). Boil and stir for another minute. Remove from the heat.

3 Stir in the margarine and vanilla. Pour into a single serving bowl or individual serving cups. Chill for 2 hours before serving.

Per serving: Calories 233 (from Fat 74); Fat 8g (Saturated 3g); Cholesterol 0mg; Sodium 255mg; Carbohydrate 38g (Dietary Fiber 2g); Protein 4g.

Baking Cakes and Pies

If you have a sweet tooth, you probably have a special place in your heart for moist cakes and right-out-of-the-oven pies. These sweet, delectable desserts are a great way to end any meal. Add a scoop of dairy-free ice cream (see the next section for some recipes) to these treats, and you may be in heaven. Even better, one of the following desserts combines the best of both worlds — the ice cream pie! These recipes replace the ice cream, milk, sour cream, and cheese with nondairy alternatives — all while not compromising on taste.

After you try these recipes, think about other favorite dessert recipes you've made in the past. Do they contain dairy ingredients? If so, using similar approaches to replacing the dairy ingredients as I show in this section, try modifying — and giving new life to — those desserts, too.

Italian Ice Cream Pie

A blend of cherries, chocolate, and rum gives this rich pie a festive appearance and flavor. This is a modern adaptation of an old Italian recipe for *tortoni*, a creamy, semi-frozen dessert.

Preparation time: *25 minutes (including time for the ice cream to soften)*

Freezing time: *1 hour*

Yield: *One 9-inch pie (8 servings)*

½ gallon vanilla nondairy ice cream

¼ cup light rum

1 tablespoon pure vanilla extract

1 small jar maraschino cherries, drained and chopped (reserve ¼ cup of the cherry juice)

6 ounces carob chips (find them at natural foods stores) or dairy-free chocolate chips

9-inch ready-made, dairy-free chocolate crumb crust

1 Leave the nondairy ice cream out at room temperature until slightly softened, about 10 minutes.

2 In a large mixing bowl, combine the nondairy ice cream, rum, vanilla, cherries, cherry juice, and carob chips. Stir with a large spoon until the ingredients are well blended and the mixture is smooth. (A stand mixer with paddle attachment is quicker and easier than mixing by hand. Chill the bowl first before mixing to keep the ice cream nice and frosty.)

3 Pour the mixture into the pie shell. Cover with foil and place in the freezer until hardened, about 1 hour. Slice and serve.

Vary It! *Instead of using vanilla nondairy ice cream, try Chocolate Tofu Ice Cream. You can find the recipe later in this chapter. In place of maraschino cherries, you also can substitute ¼ cup fresh or canned pitted cherries (any kind) and ¼ cup of their juice. (If using fresh cherries, add an extra ¼ cup of nondairy ice cream in place of the juice.)*

Per serving: *Calories 606 (from Fat 272); Fat 30g (Saturated 9g); Cholesterol 0mg; Sodium 513mg; Carbohydrate 74g (Dietary Fiber 1g); Protein 5g.*

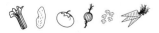

Poppy Seed Cake

This recipe was adapted from Ukrainian Poppy Seed Cake, a longtime favorite recipe from the near-and-dear-to-my-heart Moosewood Cookbook (Ten Speed Press) by Mollie Katzen. In this version, cow's milk is replaced with soymilk, and the cake is topped with a simple dusting of confectioner's sugar. The not-too-sweet cake is delicate and light in texture.

Preparation time: *30 minutes*

Cooking time: *40 minutes*

Cooling time: *1 hour and 10 minutes*

Yield: *10 servings*

¾ *cup poppy seeds*

1 cup vanilla or plain soymilk (or your choice of nondairy milk)

½ *cup nondairy, trans-fat-free margarine plus additional for greasing the pan*

1 cup sugar

3 eggs (or equivalent amount of cholesterol-free egg replacer)

2 cups flour

1 tablespoon baking powder

1 teaspoon baking soda

½ *teaspoon salt*

1 teaspoon vanilla extract

3 tablespoons lemon juice

Confectioner's sugar for dusting

1 In a small saucepan, combine poppy seeds and soymilk. Heat to just before boiling, and then remove from the heat and set aside. Let the poppy seeds soak in the milk for at least 15 minutes. Preheat the oven to 350 degrees. Use margarine to grease a 10-inch tube or bundt pan (see Figure 14-1 for an example of a bundt pan).

2 In a large mixing bowl, cream together the ½ cup of margarine and the sugar. Add the eggs and beat until smooth and creamy.

3 In a separate bowl, sift together the dry ingredients. Add the dry mixture in batches to the margarine mixture, alternating with the poppy seed and milk mixture. Stir until the ingredients are thoroughly blended. Add the vanilla and lemon juice, and then mix well.

4 Spread the batter into the prepared pan. Bake for 50 minutes, or until a toothpick inserted into the cake comes out clean.

5 Cool the cake in the pan on a cooling rack for 10 minutes, and then invert the pan and remove the cake, placing it onto a plate. Let the cake cool completely, 60 minutes. Before slicing and serving, use a strainer or sieve to dust the top of the cake with confectioner's sugar.

Per serving: Calories 340 (from Fat 139); Fat 15g (Saturated 5g); Cholesterol 64mg; Sodium 483mg; Carbohydrate 44g (Dietary Fiber 2g); Protein 7g.

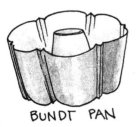

Figure 14-1: You can use a bundt pan to make your Poppy Seed Cake.

BUNDT PAN

Quick and Easy
Tofu Cherry Cheesecake

Tofu makes a fabulous replacement for cream cheese in cheesecake recipes. This cheesecake is inspired by recipes I first made with guidance from Louise Hagler in her classic *Tofu Cookery* (Book Publishing Company). You can use a ready-made, 9-inch graham cracker crust (which holds the same volume as the 8-inch springform pan used in this recipe). You may want to double the recipe for a party.

Preparation time: *30 minutes*

Cooking time: *About 30 minutes*

Chilling time: *2 hours*

Yield: *8 servings (1 pie)*

Crust

1¼ cups graham cracker crumbs

1 tablespoon sugar

⅓ cup nondairy, trans-fat-free margarine, melted

Combine the graham cracker crumbs and sugar in a medium bowl. Add the melted margarine to the crumb mixture. Stir until blended, and then press the crumbs into the bottom and sides of an 8-inch nonstick springform pan. Set aside.

Filling

1¾ 12-ounce aseptic boxes (or 1¼ pounds water-packed) firm tofu

1½ cups sugar, divided

1 teaspoon pure vanilla extract

½ teaspoon pure almond extract

⅛ teaspoon salt

One 15-ounce can cherry pie filling

1 If using water-packed tofu, remove the excess liquid from the compressed tofu (refer to Figure 14-2). If you use tofu in aseptic packaging, this step can be omitted.

2 In a blender or food processor, blend the tofu, ¼ pound at a time, with 1 cup of the sugar, adding ¼ cup sugar with each addition of tofu. Process until the ingredients are well blended.

3 Preheat the oven to 350 degrees. Pour the tofu-sugar mixture into a bowl. Mix in the vanilla and almond extracts, salt, and remaining ½ cup sugar. Blend well.

4 Pour the mixture into the graham cracker crust and bake for about 40 minutes. When the cheesecake is done, it will be slightly risen on the edges with small cracks on the surface. The middle will not have risen, but it will be springy to the touch and will have a dry, firm appearance.

5 Chill the cheesecake for at least 2 hours after baking. Top with canned cherry filling before serving.

Tip: *You can minimize cracking on the cheesecake surface by using a water bath during baking. Because it's easy for water to seep into the cheesecake, here's an alternative method that seems helpful in minimizing cracking while protecting against a soggy crust: Simply place a shallow pan filled with 2 to 3 inches of hot water into the oven on the rack beneath the cheesecake. The moisture given off by the pan of water helps to keep the cheesecake above it moist, resulting in fewer cracks in the batter as it bakes.*

Per serving: *Calories 438 (from Fat 133); Fat 15g (Saturated 4g); Cholesterol 0mg; Sodium 215mg; Carbohydrate 67g (Dietary Fiber 2g); Protein 12g.*

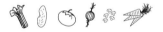

PRESSING TOFU

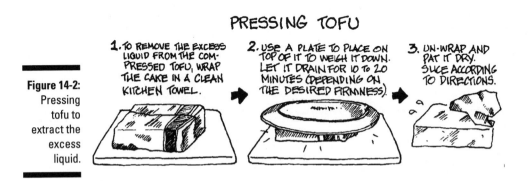

Figure 14-2: Pressing tofu to extract the excess liquid.

1. TO REMOVE THE EXCESS LIQUID FROM THE COMPRESSED TOFU, WRAP THE CAKE IN A CLEAN KITCHEN TOWEL.

2. USE A PLATE TO PLACE ON TOP OF IT TO WEIGH IT DOWN. LET IT DRAIN FOR 10 TO 20 MINUTES (DEPENDING ON THE DESIRED FIRMNESS).

3. UN-WRAP AND PAT IT DRY. SLICE ACCORDING TO DIRECTIONS.

Island Upside-Down Cake

This cake is very moist and has a wonderful soft, springy texture. The blend of bananas, pineapple, coconut, and pecans is scrumptious, and the fragrance is divine. Serve it at your next summer picnic or cookout. This nondairy version is indistinguishable from versions made with cow's milk.

Preparation time: *20 minutes*

Cooking time: *40 minutes*

Cooling time: *15 minutes*

Yield: *8 servings*

¼ cup nondairy, trans-fat-free margarine

½ cup sugar

One 20-ounce can unsweetened pineapple rings, drained (reserve the juice) (If you chose to use fresh pineapple, check Figure 14-3 for cutting and coring one.)

1 ripe banana, mashed

1 egg (or equivalent amount of cholesterol-free egg replacer)

1 cup plain or vanilla soymilk (or your choice of nondairy milk) mixed with 1½ teaspoons vinegar or fresh lemon juice

¾ cup brown sugar

½ cup sweetened, flaked coconut

⅓ cup chopped pecans

2 tablespoons vegetable oil

1 teaspoon pure vanilla extract

1¼ cups all-purpose flour

½ teaspoon baking soda

1½ teaspoons baking powder

½ teaspoon salt

1 Preheat the oven to 350 degrees. In an 8-x-8-inch stovetop-safe glass baking pan (or in a small saucepan), melt the margarine over low heat. Add the sugar, stir, and continue to cook for a few minutes until the sugar has completely dissolved into the margarine.

2 Add about 5 tablespoons of the reserved pineapple juice to the margarine and sugar mixture. Stir until completely blended, remove the pan from the heat, and set it aside. (If using a saucepan in Step 1, pour mixture into the bottom of an 8-x-8-inch baking pan.)

3 Arrange 6 pineapple rings on the bottom of the baking pan in two lines of three rings each (see Figure 14-4).

4 In a mixing bowl, combine the banana, egg, soymilk, brown sugar, coconut, pecans, oil, and vanilla. Mix until well blended and smooth. Add the flour, baking soda, baking powder, and salt. Mix until well blended and smooth.

5 Pour the batter over the pineapple rings in the baking pan. Bake for 40 minutes, or until the cake is set in the middle and lightly browned.

6 Remove the cake from the oven and cool in the pan on a cooling rack for 15 minutes. When the pan is cool enough to handle, invert the cake onto a serving plate. Cut into 8 squares and serve warm.

Per serving: *Calories 377 (from Fat 134); Fat 15g (Saturated Fat 4g); Cholesterol 0mg; Sodium 380mg; Carbohydrate 59g (Dietary Fiber 3g); Protein 4g.*

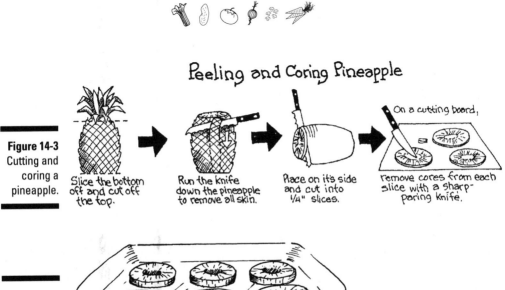

Peeling and Coring Pineapple

Figure 14-3
Cutting and coring a pineapple.

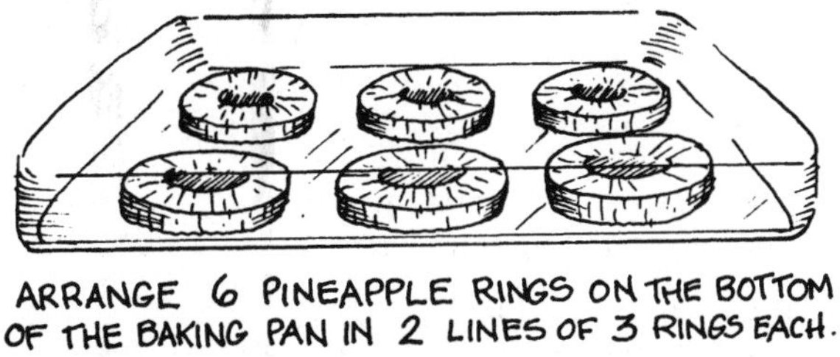

Slice the bottom off and cut off the top.

Run the knife down the pineapple to remove all skin.

Place on it's side and cut into ¼" slices.

On a cutting board, remove cores from each slice with a sharp-paring knife.

Figure 14-4
Arranging the pineapple rings.

ARRANGE 6 PINEAPPLE RINGS ON THE BOTTOM OF THE BAKING PAN IN 2 LINES OF 3 RINGS EACH.

Screaming for Ice Cream!

Nothing is as good as homemade ice cream on a hot summer day. So don't let lactose intolerance or any other detour from dairy deter you from your mission! You can make a delicious, frozen, dairy-like dessert featuring tofu as a replacement for milk and cream, two basic ingredients in homemade ice cream. The following section includes two of my all-time favorite flavors — strawberry and chocolate.

I also include two other recipes to show the range of options you have when you make nondairy ice cream from scratch. One recipe uses rice milk to make another one of my favorite flavors — mint chocolate chip. The other uses almond milk to make rich peach ice cream. Of course, you can substitute any nondairy milk — plain or vanilla — for either of these recipes.

Homemade ice cream is best after it has had several hours to sit in the freezer and harden a bit. Nondairy ice cream is no different. Ice cream fresh from the ice cream maker, without time to harden, is closer to soft-serve or a milkshake in consistency.

Strawberry Tofu Ice Cream

The flavor and texture of tofu-based ice cream is somewhat different from ice cream made with cream. It's not as creamy, and it has a slight "beany" flavor. You'll like it, though, and it can be used in all the same ways that dairy-based ice cream can be used.

Preparation time: *5 minutes*

Freezing time: *35 minutes*

Yield: *12½ servings*

Special equipment: *Ice cream maker*

16 ounces soft, silken tofu

1 cup plain or vanilla soymilk
(or your choice of nondairy milk)

1½ cups sugar

¼ cup fresh lemon juice

Two 20-ounce packages of frozen, unsweetened strawberries, semi-thawed, or 4 cups sliced fresh strawberries

2 tablespoons vanilla

¼ teaspoon salt

1 Process all the ingredients in a blender in four equal parts until smooth and creamy.

2 Freeze the mixture in a hand-operated or electric ice cream maker for approximately 35 minutes (or according to your machine's manufacturer's instructions) and serve.

Per serving: Calories 163 (from Fat 14); Fat 2g (Saturated 0g); Cholesterol 0mg; Sodium 55mg; Carbohydrate 36g (Dietary Fiber 2g); Protein 3g.

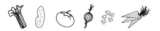

Chocolate Tofu Ice Cream

Simple and delicious. The texture of this nondairy ice cream is soft and creamy, somewhere between chocolate mousse and smooth gelato. The flavor is all chocolaty goodness.

Preparation time: *5 minutes*

Freezing time: *35 minutes*

Yield: *10 servings*

Special equipment: *Ice cream maker*

2 pounds soft, silken tofu

2 cups plain or vanilla soymilk (or your choice of nondairy milk)

2 cups sugar

½ cup unsweetened cocoa powder

2 tablespoons vanilla

¼ teaspoon salt

1 Process all the ingredients in a blender in four equal parts until smooth and creamy.

2 Freeze the mixture in a hand-operated or electric ice cream maker for approximately 35 minutes (or according to your machine's manufacturer's instructions) and serve.

Per serving: *Calories 233 (from Fat 36); Fat 4g (Saturated 1g); Cholesterol 0mg; Sodium 70mg; Carbohydrate 46g (Dietary Fiber 2g); Protein 7g.*

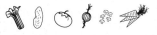

Mint Chocolate Chip Ice Cream

The minty flavor balances nicely with the rice milk in this recipe. Serve a dish with sliced bananas or inside a cantaloupe half for a refreshing summer treat.

Preparation time: *36 minutes*

Freezing time: *35 minutes*

Yield: *12 servings*

Special equipment: *Ice cream maker*

1 tablespoon arrowroot starch (available in natural foods stores)

6 cups vanilla rice milk (or your choice of nondairy milk)

1 cup sugar

3 teaspoons peppermint extract

2 teaspoons pure vanilla extract

3 drops of green food coloring (optional)

1½ cups nondairy chocolate chips (Trader Joe's brand is dairy-free)

1 Whisk the arrowroot starch into ¼ cup of the rice milk and set aside.

2 Mix the remaining rice milk and sugar in a saucepan. Cook over medium-high heat until the mixture boils, about 6 minutes. As soon as the mixture boils, take it off the heat and stir in the arrowroot mixture. Stir in the peppermint extract, vanilla extract, and food coloring (if desired). Set the mixture aside and let it cool for at least 30 minutes.

3 Freeze the mixture in a hand-operated or electric ice cream maker for approximately 35 minutes (or according to your machine's manufacturer's instructions). Add the carob chips during the last 5 to 10 minutes of freezing.

Vary It! *Around the winter holidays, replace chocolate chips with several crushed peppermint candy canes or use a combination of chocolate chips and crushed candy canes. Add a few drops of red food coloring in place of green.*

Per serving: *Calories 218 (from Fat 46); Fat 5g (Saturated 2g); Cholesterol 0mg; Sodium 33mg; Carbohydrate 43g (Dietary Fiber 0g); Protein 2g.*

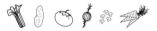

Peach Ice Cream

This ice cream tastes especially good made with fresh, locally grown peaches when they're in season. Experiment with other seasonal fresh fruits, too, including equal amounts of cantaloupe or honeydew chunks or berry mixtures.

Preparation time: *5 minutes*

Freezing time: *35 minutes*

Yield: *10 servings*

Special equipment: *Ice cream maker*

6 cups vanilla almond milk
(or your choice of nondairy milk)

3 cups peeled and sliced fresh
or frozen peaches

1 cup sugar

2 tablespoons arrowroot starch

2 teaspoons pure vanilla extract

¼ teaspoon salt

1 Process all the ingredients except peaches in a blender until smooth and creamy. Add the peaches next and pulse once or twice, creating small chunks of peach.

2 Freeze the mixture in a hand-operated or electric ice cream maker for approximately 35 minutes (or according to your machine's manufacturer's instructions) and serve.

Vary It! *For a stronger peach flavor, replace 1 cup almond milk with 1 cup peach nectar.*

Per serving: *Calories 159 (from Fat 16); Fat 2g (Saturated 0g); Cholesterol 0mg; Sodium 151mg; Carbohydrate 35g (Dietary Fiber 1g); Protein 1g.*

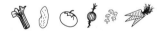

Part IV
Living — and Loving — the Dairy-Free Lifestyle

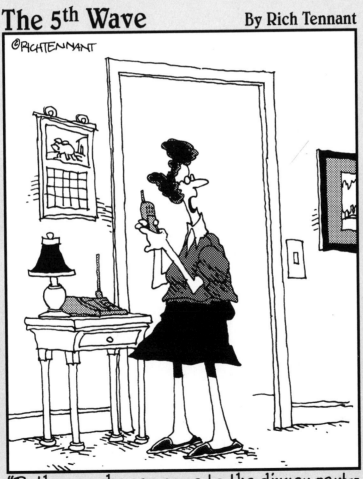

The 5th Wave   By Rich Tennant

"Beth says she can come to the dinner party, but she's allergic to cow's milk. Does that mean we can't invite your mother?"

In this part . . .

Learning to live without dairy products takes time. It requires you to acquire knowledge, master new skills, and recondition old habits. That's why, for most people, big lifestyle changes happen gradually, a step at a time.

In this part of the book, I explain what some of those steps are and describe strategies for dealing with them. I cover ideas for managing meals at home or away, including tips for sidestepping dairy ingredients at restaurants and when you travel.

I also devote several chapters to going dairy-free during different life stages. For example, if you or someone you love is pregnant and dairy-free, you may have questions about what, if any, issues you should be concerned about for mom and baby-to-be. Or maybe you're looking for detailed information and advice about raising dairy-free kids and teens. If so, you've come to the right place. Finally, I include a chapter with tips for continuing a health-supporting, dairy-free diet all the way through adulthood, particularly when you're beginning to age.

Chapter 15

Managing Social Situations

*E*ating is one of life's simple pleasures. People like to eat in the company of others in a social setting, and the kinds of foods they share when they're with friends and family form some of their dearest traditions and memories. That's why it's important to think about how best to handle social situations that involve food, especially the dairy foods you want to avoid. Some approaches are more effective than others. The trick is to stick to your dairy-free diet without spoiling your enjoyment of those meals you have with the people you love — and without hurting their feelings. You can accomplish this much easier than you may think.

In this chapter, I share some tips for getting what you need from social situations while keeping everyone in your life happy — and well fed. I cover advice on how to gracefully interact with others in a variety of settings, how to plan and prepare meals everyone in your family will love, and how to negotiate differences in food preferences in social settings at home and in other's homes.

Explaining Your Dairy-Free Diet

Your dairy-free diet doesn't have to be anyone's concern but your own. You don't owe anyone any explanation about your diet. It's even possible that some people may never find out that your diet is different — unless, of course, you tell them.

The more-likely scenario, though, is that your diet is going to be an issue at some point. If you're dairy-free, you're different. The way dairy-free diets are viewed is changing, but at this point, dairy products are still highly integrated into meals nearly everywhere you go in North America and Europe.

Because dairy-free diets aren't mainstream yet, you're the one who will likely have to do the adapting when you're in social situations. Adapting often entails telling people about your dietary restrictions and explaining why you don't do dairy. In this section, I offer some things to think about as you explain your diet to other people.

Responding to inquiring minds

You may prefer privacy and feel uncomfortable sharing personal details with people outside your closest circle of family and friends. If so, that's okay. However, realize that when it comes to your diet, you're likely to find yourself in social situations that force you to explain what you're eating — or not eating — and why. You don't have to respond when people probe, but it's easier if you can be prepared with a diplomatic response.

If someone asks about your decision to go dairy-free, the best response is a simple, straightforward answer. For example, you can say:

> "I've realized that dairy products don't agree with me, so I'm learning to replace them with other foods."

If your reasons for avoiding dairy have to do with ethical or political motivations, this isn't the time to pontificate or criticize someone else's lifestyle. Simply stick to the facts about your own eating style. Rely on your own judgment, but realize that when most people ask questions about your diet, they're just curious. The idea may be new to them, and they're exploring, not criticizing or judging.

Handling questions about your health

You may be dairy-free because you don't absorb lactose well, or it may be because you're trying to control your saturated fat intake to protect your heart. These are good reasons to avoid dairy, and people may find them interesting. After they discover that you eat a dairy-free diet for health reasons, they may begin to wonder whether they should be doing the same thing.

It's natural to be curious about other people's choices. Your diet may prompt other people to ask you questions, and some of those questions may get personal. Others may want to know how you handle certain situations and may be curious about the specifics concerning your health. They may want to know your cholesterol level so they can see how it compares with theirs. If you need some solid information to help explain the health benefits of going dairy-free, check out Chapter 2.

How you handle personal questions about your health history is up to you — you can choose to divulge or not — but do anticipate that people will ask. Understanding their motivations — that your diet may be novel to them and that it may prompt them to think about their own — may help you to feel more comfortable sharing your rationale with others who are interested.

Sharing your views gently

Your goal in presenting yourself — and your diet — to the world is to do so in a way that makes the best impression. Assuming you care what people think, I recommend an approach that will endear you to others and not put them off.

The way you talk to others about your diet choices — and the choices that other people make — has the potential of cementing or dissolving relationships. Food choices are a very personal matter, so you need to be careful about how you approach the topic with others. If you're overbearing — bossy or belligerent — you'll come off as being unstable or uncouth. If you're preachy or harsh, you'll put people off. Your diet may be healthier, and it may follow the ethical high road and the ecologically responsible path. However, you won't convince others if you hit them over the head with it.

Instead, answer questions politely, and be open to sharing your knowledge and experience when somebody cares enough to approach you for insight. Lead by example. Show others that it's possible to follow a dairy-free diet easily, deliciously, and nutritiously.

Supporting the family member who's going dairy-free

If a dairy-free member of your family finds it challenging to avoid dairy products, you can help. Consider the circumstances and come up with a plan. For example, you may decide to make a gesture of support by going dairy-free yourself when you're at home. At the very least, it may help to refrain from eating certain dairy products — ice cream, cheesy pizza, or a cheese-filled dessert, for example — when you're in the presence of the dairy-free member of your family. Be sensitive to your family member's situation and help to ease the transition to living dairy-free however you can.

Managing Family Meals

Planning and preparing family meals so that everyone is happy can sometimes be a recipe for disaster. Some food decisions are easy. Movie night? Break out the popcorn. A summertime meal? Corn on the cob and fresh, sliced tomatoes are everyone's favorites.

Other food decisions aren't as easy though. When you have a special dietary need in your family, such as when you're trying to eliminate dairy products, family meals can be a bit more challenging. For example, when you start talking about taking the cheese off the pizza or finding a substitute in which to dunk your cookies, finding a middle ground may be difficult. That's where the advice I share in this section comes into play.

Being aware of the issues you can run into and having a plan for addressing them helps you successfully manage your family relationships as you go dairy-free. Successfully managing family meals is important because food has a way of touching people's emotions; it can be a source of joy or, if not handled well, a source of conflict.

Dealing with dairy-free meals in a mixed household

When making a meal in a household where some people eat dairy and others don't, you may find yourself frustrated trying to figure out what to serve. The solution requires you to talk through the options with your family members and negotiate a solution that works for the majority of family members most of the time.

Different solutions may be appropriate at different times, too. When you're planning a meal for two or three people, it makes sense to take a "least common denominator" approach and make something that everybody can eat. On the other hand, if you're having company, and your guests aren't dairy-free, it may make sense to offer both dairy dishes and nondairy alternatives.

As you're trying to plan meals, talk through the possible solutions with everyone in the family. And think about the following possibilities you have when feeding the gang:

✔ **Whip up two meals.** If you have the extra time, you may consider creating two entree options — one with dairy and one without. Doing so isn't the most practical step to take because with most families it usually makes more sense to fix one meal that everyone can enjoy. However, in some instances, you can make one dairy item and one nondairy item without much extra work. For example, on pizza night, make one pizza as cheesy as you want and the other dairy-free.

If you're the main cook in your household and you agree to make two options, decide who prepares what. You can make mealtimes a family affair, asking family members to do different tasks to prepare the two options together.

✔ **Focus on good food.** Put some extra love into the food you prepare to help it be as appetizing as possible. If you make the food look attractive and taste good, everyone will want to eat it — even if it doesn't contain a speck of dairy. Set a vase of flowers on the table. Use a tablecloth or pretty place mats. Display food on attractive platters and use garnishes, such as fruit slices or sprigs of fresh herbs. All these special touches say "I care" and entice the family to enjoy what they're eating.

✔ **Ask everyone to be flexible.** On occasion, it may be necessary for the dairy avoider to scrape the cheese off the lasagna or eat an apple when everyone else is eating ice cream cones. It may at times also be necessary for dairy eaters to make do with nondairy dishes and products to make it easy on the family. That's especially true if someone has a dairy allergy, in which case scraping the cheese off the noodles isn't good enough.

Set those expectations upfront so that everyone is aware. It's not easy trying to accommodate multiple food preferences under the same roof. However, if everyone can try to be as flexible as possible and adapt to the circumstances when necessary, it will make things easier — and happier — for everybody.

✔ **Adopt a spirit of adventure.** Encourage everyone in the house to get involved in meal planning and shopping for nondairy alternatives like soymilk and nondairy cheese. It can be fun to experiment with foods that are new; this experimentation may even raise everyone's awareness — and interest in — healthy eating.

✔ **Go with the dairy-free least common denominator.** Choose foods that are dairy-free at their most basic states. For example, baked potatoes, green salads, and tacos are all naturally dairy-free. If you serve these alongside a range of topping options, everyone has a choice of what to add, including dairy and nondairy ingredients. For example, let the dairy-eaters add grated cheese, creamy dressings, or sour cream. Dairy-free diners instead can go with the avocado slices, plain soy yogurt, salsa, or chopped tomatoes.

The key to making a dairy-free lifestyle work in a mixed household is flexibility and a positive attitude. If you try to foster a spirit of cooperation and tolerance, the dietary differences among your family members will be easier to resolve.

If you find it difficult to reconcile the needs of the dairy eaters and dairy avoiders in your home, talk to other people who are living with similar circumstances. Surf the Web for chat groups or blogs where people share their tips for managing meals in families with members who avoid particular foods.

Negotiating which products to buy

When you live in a mixed home where some people eat dairy products and others don't, each of the household members has to help decide which products to purchase at the store. Even if everyone in your household stays away from dairy, you still have choices to make. So how do you do so?

With some products, you can purchase everyone's favorites. For example, in my home, my husband and son drink rice milk, and I drink vanilla almond milk. However, some food decisions aren't this easy. For example, it may not make sense to have more than one brand of nondairy cheese in the refrigerator if you use it so seldom that one package spoils before you can use both. That's where finding the dairy-free middle ground comes into play.

Keep the following strategies in mind to help zero in on how many dairy products — and which ones — you should buy:

- ✔ **Get everyone in your family involved.** You can have taste tests on different brands and varieties of nondairy beverages, cheeses, and other products. Make sure everyone gives an opinion about their favorites.

- ✔ **Aim for consensus.** Make a list of the dairy-free foods that everyone can agree that they like. Go through each category — breakfast foods, soups, salads, sides, main dishes, dips and spreads, breads, snacks, and desserts. Peruse the recipe chapters in Part III to start the discussion. After you identify the foods that everyone likes, you can make those foods more often.

When a consensus isn't possible, rotate products so that everyone gets their favorite once in a while.

Getting the whole family involved

One great strategy for gaining buy-in for meals is to give others a hand in planning and preparing them. That's especially true of children. If you can get your kids involved in preparing the nondairy meal, they'll be more likely to eat it. I talk about getting kids involved in more detail in Chapter 18.

Dinnertime is a convenient time to focus on getting others involved. This is true because the meal is a little less rushed than breakfast, and family members are more likely to be home. Use the opportunity to give kids a few tasks related to planning and preparing dairy-free entrees.

For example, younger kids can go to the cupboard or refrigerator to get supplies, and they may be able to perform other simple tasks such as dumping grated nondairy cheese into a pot. Older kids can help with assembling sandwiches or setting the table. They also may be able to perform other tasks with supervision, such as stirring food on the stovetop or removing a cheeseless pizza from the oven.

Keeping meals simple

Even when all members have different food preferences or tolerances, family meals don't have to be complicated. After all, how many families do you know in which every member eats exactly the same foods? Probably not many.

The key is to keep in mind the importance of taking a *participatory approach*. This approach requires you to ensure that each family member gets a chance to express his or her interests and preferences, to talk openly about the options, and to make sure everyone feels they have a say in the decisions. And you must negotiate to keep it simple.

In most families, simplifying meals means agreeing on a few staple products to keep on hand, figuring out which foods make sense to buy in more than one brand or variety, and honing in on a lineup of favorite meals that most of you enjoy most of the time. Doing these things makes planning meals easier and less time consuming. It also will help you save money by cutting waste.

Enjoying popular nondairy meals

You can maximize your family's satisfaction with nondairy meals by making their favorites — often. Some tried-and-true options are so good that family members aren't likely to notice that they're dairy-free. Some of the following suggestions are good places to start because they let individual family members customize their meals:

✔ **Put together a taco or burrito bar.** Set out flour and corn tortillas and lots of fillings, and let everyone assemble their own dairy-free tacos or burritos. Good fillings to add to the line up include mashed avocado, nondairy grated cheese, black beans, refried beans, nondairy sour cream, chopped tomatoes and lettuce, black olives, mashed sweet potatoes, and your favorite salsa.

✔ **Serve pasta with nondairy toppings.** Dish up pasta tossed with marinara sauce and topped with nondairy Parmesan cheese. For a change of pace, vary the shape of the noodles. You also can toss pasta with olive oil and chopped garlic instead of using a tomato-based pasta sauce. If you go this route, you can add steamed vegetables or sautéed spinach or other greens. Provide extra toppings, such as pesto, sundried tomatoes, black olives, and chopped walnuts, on the side so family members can add them if they so choose.

✔ **Provide a baked potato bar.** Similar to the taco and burrito bar, a baked potato bar allows family members to customize their baked potatoes. Good tater toppings include chopped steamed broccoli, salsa, nondairy sour cream, guacamole, black olives, grated nondairy cheese, chopped tomatoes and lettuce, and thick lentil soup. The brown gravy served with the creamed potatoes recipe in Chapter 10 also is good on a baked potato.

✔ **Offer a salad bar.** By now, you probably get the idea. Do the same thing you did with the tacos, burritos, pasta, and potatoes, but focus on cold nondairy toppings. Examples include chopped bell peppers, tomatoes, cucumbers, black olives, sliced strawberries, croutons, garbanzo beans, sunflower seeds, raisins, sliced almonds, grated carrots, minced green onions, and sliced radishes. Vary the greens — spinach, Romaine, spring mix — and offer a variety of nondairy salad dressings from which to choose.

Check out the recipes in Part III for more dairy-free family meal ideas.

Hosting Dairy Eaters in Your Dairy-Free Home

Having guests in your home can be especially challenging if you're living dairy-free. Unless your guests also are dairy-free, they're likely to be unfamiliar with some of the nondairy products you may be routinely eating in place of other common dairy products. They may, for example, expect to see cow's milk in your refrigerator, not almond milk. And they may find cheeseless pizza a bit odd.

So, in this section, I offer a few suggestions for times when you may have dairy-eaters staying at your home for more than one meal. You'll find this advice helpful whether you have company for a weekend or longer.

Providing options

Offering choices is always a good idea when hosting visitors. Approach entertaining guests using some of the same strategies you'd use with your family. One way is to offer meals that include a range of options for customizing each dish. In the earlier section "Enjoying popular nondairy meals," I offer some suggestions for meals that lend themselves to customization.

Before they arrive, ask your guests about their food likes and dislikes to get a feel for how easy or challenging it may be to come up with meal ideas you can all enjoy. To the extent possible, try to identify nondairy options that everybody already likes. I provide some suggestions in the next section.

When all else fails, assume you may need to have both nondairy and dairy food options at home while you have guests. For example, you may find it makes sense to keep a half gallon of cow's milk alongside the carton of rice milk for the duration. That's okay. Do what makes sense for your situation.

Serving foods where dairy isn't the star

In addition to the flexible meal options I list earlier in the chapter, you can experiment with other meal ideas that your guests may enjoy. Because many ethnic cuisines are largely or entirely dairy-free, look to other parts of the world for inspiration.

You'll find recipes for some ethic dairy-free dishes in Part III of this book. Good examples include Indonesian Saté and West African Peanut Soup. Other excellent options include the following:

- ✔ **Chinese cuisine:** Dairy products are nearly nonexistent in Asian cuisine. A wide variety of stir-fried meals incorporate rice, vegetables, tofu, meats, and nondairy seasonings.

- ✔ **Japanese cuisine:** Options include many varieties of sushi and *tempura* (vegetables or seafood dipped in a nondairy batter and lightly fried in oil).

- ✔ **Middle Eastern cuisine:** Dishes you may want to try include hummus, *falafel* (deep-fried balls made from ground garbanzo beans) served in pita pockets, *fattoush* (a chopped green salad that includes toasted pieces of pita bread), and curried couscous salad made with saffron, raisins, slivered almonds, orange zest, onion, and spices.

Thumb through ethnic cookbooks to get other ideas, and surf the Web for hundreds of recipes to try.

Being a Gracious Guest

When someone invites you to his home for a meal, it's often to commemorate a happy occasion. Having special dietary needs may complicate matters. Should you tell your host that you can't eat dairy? If so, how should you make your needs known? And if you don't divulge your needs, what happens when the main course turns out to be pasta with Alfredo sauce? This situation turns out bad for everyone — the guest goes hungry, and the host feels terrible and embarrassed. So, in this section, I discuss these and other aspects of being — and remaining — a welcome guest.

Telling your host about your needs

Sharing your dietary needs with your host is nothing to be ashamed of. In fact, if you're open about your needs, you may find you're not alone. Many people have special dietary preferences or restrictions because of health issues or personal preferences. They're watching their saturated fat or cholesterol, or they're limiting added sugars because of diabetes. Maybe they're cutting down on salt to control their blood pressure. Or maybe they're vegetarians or *vegans,* which are vegetarians who eat no animal products whatsoever — not even eggs or dairy products.

Put yourself in the place of your host. If you had someone coming over for dinner and they didn't eat dairy products, wouldn't you want to know ahead of time? You'd want to fix a meal your guest could eat and would enjoy. You'd be disappointed if he or she didn't eat what you fixed, right? More than likely, your host would feel the same and would prefer to know.

Mention your diet at the time of the invitation. Doing so gives you an opportunity to explain exactly what you can and can't eat, and it will give your host time to plan. If the invitation is less direct — it comes in the mail or through a second party, such as a friend or your partner — you have a couple of choices, which I describe in the following sections.

Say nothing and eat what you can

If you stay silent, you'll be in the position of arriving at your host's home and making do with what's served. If the meal is a buffet or potluck with lots of different foods available, you may have plenty of dairy-free choices. In that case, you can load up your plate with foods you can eat, and no one may notice that you skipped the cheese strata.

If you decide to take this route, be sure to have a substantial snack beforehand just in case you can't find enough dairy-free foods to fill yourself up.

Contact the host and tell her about your diet restrictions

Give the host a call, thank her for the invitation, and then explain that you have some special dietary considerations. Tell your host that you wanted to mention your diet so she didn't go to any trouble serving something you couldn't eat. At the same time, you may tell your host that she needn't go to any special effort on your behalf.

Here's an example of a gracious way of broaching the issue with your host:

> "Thanks so much for the wonderful dinner invitation. I'm really looking forward to coming! By the way, I should tell you that I can't eat dairy products. Please don't feel you have to fix anything special for me. I'm sure I'll find plenty to eat. I just didn't want you to go to the trouble of fixing something for me that I couldn't eat."

Most likely your host will ask you some questions to help better understand what you can and can't eat. It's polite to answer honestly. If he says he was planning to serve a green salad with golden beets, sugared pecans, dried cranberries, and goat cheese, tell him that sounds great. You can have the same thing — minus the cheese. Simple enough.

If it's not that simple, help your host troubleshoot some solutions. Find out what else he plans to serve — you may be fine with nothing more than side dishes.

Contact the host and offer to bring a dish

This option works well when the setting is casual and you're among people you know well. Potluck dinners and meals among friends, for example, may be good opportunities to bring a dairy-free dish you can share.

Bringing your own dish is less appropriate in formal settings. It can look pretty tacky to show up at a wedding reception or formal dinner party with a covered dish in your hands.

Assess the situation, and if appropriate, make the offer. If your host sounds worried or unsure about how to handle your diet, you may say something like:

> "Why don't you let me bring my famous dairy-free Spinach and Mushroom Manicotti? It works as an entree, and it would go well with your baked chicken."

If your host declines, don't push. You've offered. You can weigh your other options in that case. You may decide to make do with what you can eat once you get to your host's home (and eat a snack before leaving home, just in case), or you may be able to eat very small portions of dairy foods, depending on your level of intolerance or your personal convictions.

Making do if your host's meal doesn't fit your needs

Despite your best intentions, sometimes you can't give your host a warning before you arrive for dinner (or he may forget or do a poor job of meeting your needs). If that happens, plan ahead and have a strategy in mind — just in case.

Imagine this worst-case scenario: You arrive at dinner, and you sit down to eat. The choices include a salad tossed with grated cheese, a cheese-infused casserole, broccoli with cheese sauce, and baked custard for dessert. If you encounter this situation, eat what you can. Eat around the dairy. Scrape it off, scoop food from an area not coated in cheese — be creative — but try to avoid looking pitiful with nothing more than a dinner roll on your plate. Make your plate look as full as you can. (Remember the old trick from childhood? Spread the food around.) You won't starve. You can always supplement with a snack when you get home.

Whatever you do, don't get angry and make a fuss that you can't find anything to eat. Otherwise, you can ruin the meal by spoiling everyone's good time and never be welcomed back.

If you know you're going someplace where the choices may be slim, have a snack before you leave home. That way, you won't find yourself gnawing on your knuckles if there isn't much you can eat. Another option: Fill up on other nondairy items, including appetizers like crackers and veggies that may come before the meal.

Chapter 16

Dodging Dairy on the Mooove: Eating Out

*E*ating out when you're dairy-free poses a different set of challenges than those you face at home. Eating meals at home has the distinct advantage of giving you maximum control over what you eat. When you're at home, you get to choose the ingredients that go into each dish, and you have access to food labels and can read what's in the food you buy. Not so when you're away from home.

Eating out requires special effort on your part to successfully avoid dairy ingredients in foods. In this chapter, I offer some good-sense advice about how to steer clear of dairy products when you eat out at restaurants. I include information on deciding where to eat, examining the menu, working with restaurant personnel, and making good choices to maximize your enjoyment without jeopardizing your diet. Beyond restaurants, I also cover other travel situations that may necessitate special arrangements to ensure that you get what you need.

Maintaining a Positive Attitude

Eating out is meant to be fun, so don't let your dairy-free diet get in the way. The key to staying dairy-free without spoiling your enjoyment when you're eating out is to keep things in perspective and to remain optimistic. That includes taking steps to help ensure that you have as many options as possible wherever you go.

Dairy-free friendly? Using the Internet to research restaurants

The Internet is an excellent tool for doing research on restaurants before you head out to eat. At the very least, most restaurants have a Web site where you can view menus to get a feel for how many nondairy options you may find when you get there.

Check out www.godairyfree.org for a list of dairy-free menu options at restaurants, especially in Canada. Other Web sites, such as www.veganeatingout.com and www.vegdining.com, provide information about vegan — and therefore, dairy-free — restaurant options as well.

In this section, I explain how your attitude and the way you approach eating out can add to your enjoyment when you're away from home — and make your dairy-free diet a success.

Preplanning: Why it's so important

Part of staying positive includes being proactive about making sure dairy-free dining options are available to you when you eat out. Planning ahead is a fundamental step in successfully making the transition to a dairy-free diet.

Before you go out to eat, give some thought to the circumstances in which you're likely to find yourself. Thinking about how you'll handle your meal before you leave your house may help make the process smoother after you reach the restaurant. A few questions to consider include

- ✔ **Will you be eating out with a group?** If so, be sure to voice some suggestions for restaurants. If you have some say over the choice of the restaurant, you may have a better chance of landing at an establishment that can cater to your dietary needs. For example, you're likely to find more nondairy options at a Chinese restaurant than at a pancake house.

- ✔ **What can you do to help prepare for the meal options you'll have when you eat out?** Give some forethought to what you may be able to order. If necessary, phone ahead and ask about potential options. Finer restaurants are more likely to be able to accommodate special requests because they make your food to order instead of serving foods that are premade.

- ✔ **What will you order?** If you know where you'll be eating ahead of time, you may be able to study the menu before you leave your house. Many restaurants post their menus online where you can study the options and even call ahead to make a special request.

> ✔ **Should you grab a snack before you leave home?** If it looks like you won't have many choices where you'll be eating, you always can eat something before you leave home. That way, you can order something light, enjoy the company, and not worry about going hungry. It's not likely to come to this, but it's always an option to keep up your sleeve.

Staying flexible

People who successfully stick to a dairy-free diet when they eat out share a characteristic in common — they're able to adapt to whatever environment they find themselves in. However, rolling with the punches is sometimes easier to do than it is at other times. It may be easier to be flexible when you're by yourself, for example, and more difficult when you have to keep young children happy with their meals — especially when they're hungry!

Staying flexible requires having a positive attitude. Cultivate that state of mind, and you'll find it's much easier to endure life's little bumps and turns in the road. At times when you're hungry and nondairy options are difficult to find, it helps to know that other meals will be in your future.

The important thing to keep in mind is that the occasion and your companions are more important than the food when you go out to eat. Savor the beautiful setting, the great atmosphere, the lively music, or the laughter and chatter of the people you're with. You'll have a chance to eat another, better, dairy-free meal later.

Picking the Restaurant

Where you choose to eat can have a big impact on how easy it is to eat out dairy-free. Some restaurants have more choices than others, and some restaurants are more likely than others to be able to accommodate special requests. In this section, I help you make better choices when selecting a restaurant for your next meal. I describe the pitfalls — and opportunities — for eating dairy-free at various types of restaurants.

Although you may have more control at certain times over where you go to eat and how many dairy-free choices are available when you get there, sometimes you may still end up at the Dairy Barn. When you do, your ability to make do — even if that means ordering French fries and a drink while everyone else enjoys their ice cream cones — can get you through and enable you to enjoy the occasion and the company you're with. You can compensate later by eating a big salad and a piece of fresh fruit when you get home.

Fine-dining and locally-run restaurants versus chain and fast-food establishments

When you eat out today, you have many options. You can solicit the local family diner down the street that has been owned by the same family for 20 years; you can run through the drive-through at a fast-food restaurant for a quick bite to eat; you can go with familiarity and eat at any number of chain sit-down restaurants; or you can settle in for a relaxing meal at a fine-dining establishment. When making this decision with a dairy-restricted diet, you have to pay special attention to the different menu items available for you to eat.

The advantage to eating at finer restaurants — as well as family-run restaurants — is that they're more often in a position to accommodate special requests. So, for the greatest degree of flexibility and likelihood that you may order foods that are dairy-free, seek out finer restaurants or better family restaurants. These establishments are more likely to prepare your food at the time you order it, so there's an opportunity for you to ask them to hold the cheese sauce or leave the mozzarella off the baked ziti.

In contrast, chain and fast-food restaurants are more likely to serve ready-made foods. Restaurants that cater to the masses often serve foods that were prepared and shipped — frozen — to the restaurant for reheating at the time of service. There's no opportunity to change the basic ingredients. Or, these restaurants may prepare large batches of salad, sides, and main dishes ahead of time. Once again, this situation makes it difficult (or impossible) to remove the Parmesan cheese, milk, cream sauce, or mozzarella coating before serving you.

If you're eating at a chain or fast-food restaurant, you can still adapt, however. Take a look at Table 16-1 for some common menu items and examples of ways to order them so they're dairy-free.

Table 16-1	Menu-Item Alternatives
Instead of This:	*Ask for This:*
Nachos with cheese	Nachos minus the cheese (and no sour cream)
Fettuccine Alfredo	Fettuccine with marinara sauce
Loaded baked potato	Baked potato minus the cheese and sour cream (ask for a side of salsa instead)
Caesar salad	Salad without Parmesan cheese and creamy dressing
Greek salad	Salad without feta cheese
French onion soup	Onion soup minus the melted cheese on top

Vegetarian, vegan, and natural foods options

For a wide range of dairy-free menu options, one of your best bets is to go with a natural foods, vegetarian, or vegan restaurant. These places cater to people with special dietary needs, especially those that involve avoidance of dairy products.

Natural foods stores often have little cafes tucked away in corners of their stores. At these cafes, you can sample a wide range of high-quality foods prepared with ingredients sold in the store. Some of those cafes are run in conjunction with a natural foods deli counter, where you can buy prepared salads, soups, sides, and entrees to take out or eat in.

Cafes and deli counters at natural foods stores are a great place to sample nondairy cheese, nondairy milk, and other specialty products to help you decide which brands, varieties, or flavors you like best. That way, when you go to buy these products for your home, you'll be able to take some of the guesswork out of choosing.

Vegetarian and vegan restaurants often serve many of the same products that you'll find at natural foods cafes and delis, including a wide range of non-dairy choices to accommodate vegetarians and *vegans* (vegetarians who eat no meat, fish, poultry, eggs, and dairy products).

If you eat at a vegetarian, vegan, or natural foods restaurant, you can rest assured that any menu choice marked "vegan" will be dairy-free. Some common, dairy-free menu choices at these restaurants include:

- Bean chili topped with grated nondairy cheese
- Frozen desserts made with nondairy ingredients
- Nondairy cream soup
- Pudding made with nondairy milk
- Smoothies with no dairy ingredients
- Soy lattes
- Tofu lasagna
- Veggie burger with nondairy cheese
- Veggie wrap sandwich (no dairy)
- Whole-wheat pasta primavera (no dairy)

Eateries that serve ethnic cuisine

Because most of the world's adults have some level of lactose malabsorption or intolerance, it may not surprise you to discover that they also have plenty of dairy-free food traditions. Parts of the world that are most affected include Asia and Africa as well as many parts of Latin America, the Middle East, and Mediterranean. If you have access to ethnic restaurants where you live or travel, you'll likely find lots of good-tasting, dairy-free menu choices.

At Italian restaurants, try any of the following:

✔ Antipasto (no cheese)

✔ Espresso

✔ Italian bread with olive oil for dipping

✔ Italian ice

✔ Lentil soup

✔ Minestrone soup

✔ Mixed greens salads

✔ Pasta e fagioli (pasta with beans)

✔ Pasta primavera

✔ Pizza (ask for it cheeseless)

✔ Spaghetti with marinara sauce

At Mexican restaurants, try:

✔ *Chalupas,* which are fried tortillas layered with beans, lettuce, tomatoes, and guacamole (hold the cheese and sour cream)

✔ *Churros,* a fried pastry snack

✔ Fried plantains

✔ Mixed greens salads

✔ Nachos (minus the cheese and sour cream)

✔ Spinach enchiladas (no cheese)

✔ Tacos and burritos (minus the cheese and sour cream)

✔ Tortilla chips with salsa

At Mexican and Italian restaurants, cheese often is added to foods, even if it isn't mentioned on the menu. Be sure to tell your waitperson that you don't want cheese on the item you order, even if you don't expect that food to come with cheese. At Mexican restaurants, it's a good idea to mention that you also don't want sour cream.

At Chinese restaurants, try these items:

- Almond tea
- Dumplings
- Family-style tofu or Buddha's delight
- Fried rice
- Fruit desserts
- Hot and sour soup
- Lo mein
- Minced vegetables wrapped in lettuce
- Sesame noodles
- Spring rolls and egg rolls
- Stir-fry with rice
- Sweet and sour cabbage salad
- Vegetable soup

Chinese restaurants are even more likely than vegetarian or natural foods restaurants to have many dairy-free choices available. Few, if any, menu choices at Chinese restaurants contain milk, cheese, or other dairy ingredients.

At Indian restaurants, try the following:

- Dal (lentil soup)
- Chapati, pappadam, naan, and roti (Indian breads)
- Curries with steamed rice
- *Halwa,* a dense, flour- or nut-based dessert cut into small cubes
- Lentil, chickpea, chicken, and vegetable entrees
- Samosas and pakoras (vegetable-filled appetizers)

At Indian restaurants, where names of foods may be unfamiliar to you, tell the waitperson that you can't eat dairy products and ask whether milk, cheese, or butter are added to menu items you're interested in ordering. These ingredients may be in the foods, even if they're not mentioned on the menu. One example is *ghee,* or clarified butter, added to many foods in Indian restaurants.

At Ethiopian restaurants, try:

- Fresh vegetable salads
- *Injera,* which is large, flat, round spongy bread (you tear off small pieces and use it to pinch bits of food with your fingers from a communal plate)

- Lentil, bean, and vegetable-based dishes served directly on a sheet of injera on a tray or platter
- Various meat entrees

At Middle Eastern restaurants, try:

- Baba ghanouj (eggplant dip or appetizer)
- Dolmades (stuffed grape leaves)
- Falafel plate or sandwich (fried garbanzo bean patties; no yogurt sauce)
- Halvah (sesame dessert)
- Hummus
- Lentil soup
- Ramadan (cooked, dried fruit with nuts; no cream)
- Spinach salad (no cheese)
- Tabbouleh salad (wheat salad)

Studying the Menu

Sooner or later, you're going to end up eating at a restaurant where the dairy-free choices aren't obvious. The menu is the first resource you can study to determine whether the food you want to eat has dairy in it.

The ingredients in the menu items may be cloaked in terms that have their origins in foreign languages or culinary jargon that you aren't familiar with. If you don't know what a dish's ingredients are, the best piece of advice I have for you is to ask. Doing so is particularly smart when the menu descriptions aren't clear whether dairy ingredients have been added to the foods.

In this section, I help you get started by sharing some key points as you study the menu and what to do after you find dairy.

Doing some investigative work

When you're in an unfamiliar restaurant, you need to be able to put on your sleuth hat and figure out what ingredients are in the different dishes available. It's helpful to develop some investigative skills and strategies that you can apply to understanding restaurant menus.

Some sources of dairy are obvious. Milk and cream, whipped cream, melted or grated cheese, and cream sauces, for example, are relatively easy to spot on the menu or on your plate. Others may be subtler, though. It may be more difficult to pinpoint these more minor sources of dairy. So, depending on your level of dairy intolerance, you may need to go a step further in determining whether certain foods contain dairy ingredients.

One way to identify hidden dairy is to be sensitive to clues you can pick up on by yourself. For example, pay attention to the words used to describe menu items. Words like "creamy," "cheesy," "buttery," "au gratin," and "Alfredo" are hints that cream, milk, or cheese are likely added to menu items. (In case you're curious, "au gratin" is a food preparation term of French origin that usually infers that grated cheese is an ingredient in the top crust of a casserole or vegetable *gratin*.)

If you're sensitive to even small amounts of dairy ingredients in foods, it may be necessary for you to ask the restaurant wait staff to check package labels in the kitchen for small amounts of dairy ingredients that may be present in the supplies they use. Check out the "Working with the Wait Staff" section later in this chapter for more specific suggestions.

Different dishes may have different dairy sources, so keep a vigilant eye open. The following sections look at different courses and how dairy can pop up and what you do can to avoid it by investigating the menu.

Sleuthing into appetizers, salads, and sides

As you survey the menu and look at the listings for appetizers, salads, and sides, pay particular attention to items that may have cheese added. Many dips and stuffed items — spinach and artichoke dip and stuffed mushrooms, tomatoes, and other vegetables — are made with soft cheeses that may be grated on or melted into these menu items.

Salads, too, often have grated cheese tossed into them. Or they may be served with crumbles or round pieces of goat cheese, feta cheese, Gorgonzola, or other salad-type cheeses. Salads also may come to the table already tossed with cream-based dressings. Side dishes, such as mashed potatoes, creamed spinach, or creamed corn may have milk or cream added to maintain a creamy texture.

Opting for main dishes: Which are best?

The advice in the preceding section on appetizers, salads, and sides applies to main dishes as well. And most importantly, if you aren't sure, ask your waitperson what's in the food.

Layers of cheese often are added to entrees such as strata, lasagna, eggplant Parmesan, and casseroles. Some meat dishes also include layers of melted cheese. Examples include veal Parmesan and chicken *cordon bleu.* Club sandwiches and Monte Cristo sandwiches often contain cheese layers, too. And some dishes are smothered in cream sauce.

The best dairy-free choices usually are foods that are prepared relatively plainly — grilled meats, fish, and poultry — as well as salads and pasta dishes that are made to order and can be modified to exclude the cream or cheese.

Some of the healthiest dairy-free entree choices are listed in the earlier section "Eateries that serve ethnic cuisine." These are the vegetable-based choices common in many parts of the world. They're easy to order, too, because most of them were dairy-free from the start and don't have to be modified to remove dairy ingredients.

Enjoying desserts

Dairy products are a mainstay in restaurant desserts. There are pies and brownies *a la mode* (with ice cream!). There's the whipped cream on the berries and pie. And then there are the cream pies, ice cream sundaes, gelato, puddings, custards, crème brûlée, and cheesecakes, which all contain dairy. Many after-dinner liqueurs do as well. If you've got a sweet tooth, what should you do? Don't worry. You have options.

Tasty dairy-free dessert choices include

- Bowl of fresh berries
- Dairy-free sorbet or Italian ice
- Espresso or coffee with vanilla syrup (or another flavor)
- Fruit cobbler or crisp
- Fruit pies — apple, cherry, blueberry, or peach
- Vegan chocolate cake

Making simple substitutions

When you do find dairy ingredients in menu items, determine whether the restaurant can prepare those foods without dairy or with alternative ingredients. For example, if ice cream is added to the top of the brownie before it's served, ask whether sliced strawberries or bananas may be available instead. (This assumes, of course, that you can handle the likely small amount of milk that may be present in the brownie!) Or if you see that the pasta of the day is tossed with cream sauce, ask whether a simple olive oil and garlic dressing can be used in its place.

Get some ideas about what the alternatives may be by surveying the other items listed on the menu. You may be able to determine whether certain ingredients used on other plates can be substituted in a dish you'd like to order. For example, if you see that applesauce comes with the potato pancakes at breakfast, you may be able to ask for it over your gingerbread instead of the whipped cream that usually comes with it.

Working with the Wait Staff

When you eat out, your server can be a great advocate and can help you stay away from dairy items. So be kind and pleasant with him or her. How you present yourself, your attitude, and your confidence level may influence your success at getting what you need when you eat out. When you have special dietary needs, these factors become important in your relationships with the wait staff. The following sections give you some advice on the best ways to develop a good relationship with your server.

Being assertive (but kind)

Right from the beginning, you want to be clear about what you need when you go out to eat. You need to tell the wait staff exactly what you can and can't eat. Doing so requires you to be assertive. You need to let your waitperson know at the outset that you want to order a meal without dairy products.

Make sure you're clear and explain the types of ingredients you want to avoid. Tell the person whether you're limited to obvious sources of milk, cream, and cheese, or whether you're someone who can't even tolerate minor amounts of dairy ingredients in, for example, a piece of bread or a slice of cake.

Be explicit and give some examples of the kinds of foods you can't eat. For example, you may say something like this:

> "I really have to be careful, because I'm very sensitive to even small amounts of dairy products. If there's cream in the mashed potatoes or milk mixed into the mayonnaise in the coleslaw, I can't eat it."

If the server acts wishy-washy and isn't sure about whether a menu item has dairy in it or not, don't take any risks. Ask to speak to a manager. The manager has direct access to recipes and can verify whether something has dairy in it. It's better to be safe than sorry.

Flashing a smile and remaining friendly

In the preceding section, I tell you that you must be assertive when communicating with your server. However, don't be so assertive that you turn him or her off from helping you. A friendly face will get you much further. In fact, when you're asking for special attention at a restaurant, a smile and a thank you go a long way (for you and for others who will follow in your footsteps).

Restaurant personnel will be more receptive to your requests if you're pleasant in your interactions with them. If you're having trouble finding something you can eat, they'll be more likely to make suggestions and extend some extra effort on your behalf as well.

Here's a tip about tipping. If the server gives you good service, make sure you tip him or her 15 to 20 percent, especially if you've asked for several substitutions and special food items. The wait staff usually receives a pittance for an hourly wage; the majority of income comes from tips. Reward good service when you get it.

Traveling Dairy-Free

You have even less control over your meals when you're traveling than when you eat out at restaurants in familiar territory. A variety of factors can compound the challenges of getting dairy-free meals. For example, consider the following:

- **Your schedule may limit your choices.** If you check into your hotel after hours, restaurants in the area may be closed, and room service may have ended. Your only food outlet may be a vending machine or those airline peanuts you were saving.

- **Food kiosks found in airports and hotels have limited menus.** Kiosks may not carry the same range of menu items that full-service restaurants carry. They also may rely on more preprepared foods shipped in from outside kitchens, giving you less leeway for making dairy-free substitutions.

- **You don't have the home court advantage.** In your own neighborhood, you may have favorite restaurants where the staff members know you and you know the menu so well that you have no trouble getting what you need. When you're away from home, your restaurant experiences may be hit or miss.

In this section, I go into more detail about ways to increase the odds that you'll find satisfying, dairy-free foods when you travel. I include information regarding road trips, flights, and cruises.

Eating on the road

When you travel by car or bus, you're typically limited to meals at whatever happens to be near the next exit off the highway. So you're likely looking at chain restaurants, truck stops, fast-food joints, and the occasional mom-and-pop restaurant. Menus tend to be limited at these types of places; and the option to have your food made to order is unlikely. If you happen to travel by train, your choices are likely to be equally limited — or more so. Even long-haul trains with meal service tend to have limited menus. So what do you do?

One option is to map out your car trip so you hit restaurants that you know have nondairy choices on the menus. By doing your research and planning your route ahead of time, you should have food choices available to you.

Your best bet, though, may be to take matters into your own hands and carry food with you to eat on the road. That way, you have more control over what's available to you. You won't go hungry because you'll at least have a few things with you to munch on. (You also can scope out the limited menus using the tips I provide earlier in this chapter.)

What you bring depends, in part, on how long you'll be gone and whether it's convenient to bring along a cooler for perishable foods. Also consider that, depending on where you spend the night, you may have access to a refrigerator in your motel room where you can store anything you didn't eat in the car or bus that day.

If you choose to pack your own supplies, you have lots of easy and tasty choices. Here are some ideas:

- ✔ Bagels with nondairy cream cheese
- ✔ Dried fruit and nut mixtures
- ✔ Fresh fruit (apples and pears travel well without getting mushy)
- ✔ Homemade muffins, cookies, and quick breads
- ✔ Hummus and pita bread
- ✔ Individual aseptic cartons of soymilk
- ✔ Instant soup cups and oatmeal
- ✔ Peanut butter and other dairy-free sandwiches
- ✔ Peeled carrots and celery with nondairy salad dressing dips
- ✔ Small cans or aseptic boxes of fruit juice
- ✔ Soy pudding cups
- ✔ Soy yogurt
- ✔ Whole-grain crackers and tortilla chips with salsa

Don't forget to bring along disposable spoons and napkins. Small freezer packs can be refrozen in the freezer compartment of motel room refrigerators when you stop for the night. And you can fill up your cooler the next day from the hotel's ice maker. Stop at a supermarket for fresh supplies when you need them.

Flying dairy-free

Airline food service is much more limited today than it was in years past. As a result, fewer options are available for people with special dietary needs. Plus, finding appropriate food while flying is difficult because fewer airlines serve free food. Flights that used to include a full meal or snack often serve nothing now; if they do serve something, you have a limited number of selections available at high prices. What's a dairy-free traveler to do?

When you fly, it's a good idea to consider the same advice I give to people taking road trips: Bring some food from home. At the very least, bring along several portable snacks — granola bars, dried fruit and nuts, and a couple of apples — to hold you over in case you have to miss a meal and are hungry.

Solid foods generally are fine to take through security at airports, but leave drinks at home. Airlines restrict most fluids from going through security. However, you can buy water and other beverages once you've cleared security.

On longer trips, when you know you'll be served a meal, put in a request with the airline in advance for a special meal. You need to set this up with the airline's reservations desk a minimum of 24 hours before your flight, or you may be able to make the request at the time that you book your reservation. (However, keep in mind that you may not be able to make this request online.) If you do request a special meal in advance of your flight, ask the reservations agent what your options are. Airlines have cut back on the number of different special meal options they offer. Vegan meals are still available on most airlines. Because this form of vegetarian diet excludes all animal products, it's a good choice for anyone living dairy-free. Some airlines may designate this choice, "Vegetarian — no dairy."

If you miss your flight or have to take a different flight with short notice, it's likely that your special meal request will not carry over to your new flight. Be prepared by having some snack foods tucked away in case you need them.

After you've boarded your flight, take some precautions to make sure you get the meal you ordered. On most flights, the crew has a list of passengers who have ordered special meals. Check in with the flight attendants early, before the meal is served, to let them know that you're expecting a special meal.

This check-in is especially important if you're sitting at the back of the plane. It's not uncommon for special meals to be given away before they reach the back of the plane. It's not supposed to happen, but it does. Tickets can be difficult to read, and your name may be obscured. If someone ahead of you asks for a meal like the one you ordered, the flight attendant may hand it off without realizing he's giving away your meal.

Dairy-free at sea

In contrast to other forms of travel, cruise ships are more like full-service restaurants. If you're eating a dairy-free diet, your chances of getting what you need when you're cruising are similar to when you eat out at many fine restaurants.

An added advantage to eating on cruise ships is that many meals are served buffet style. That allows you to pick and choose from a wide range of items. Because you can see the finished dish before you take it, it's also likely you'll catch obvious sources of dairy, such as cheese sauce on the broccoli or grated cheese in the salad.

My story with a dairy-free lifestyle

My first job was at the neighborhood dairy, where I became an expert ice cream cone scooper and sundae maker. With parents from Wisconsin — the cheese state — all forms of milk were staples from the time I could remember.

However, my strong relationship with dairy ended in the late 1980s. By then, I'd been a vegetarian for nearly 15 years. Even though I included dairy products in my diet, I was intrigued by stories from other vegetarians who had removed dairy products from their diets and felt much better as a result. Some of these folks said they got sick less frequently. No scientific studies were available to back up the claims, but my curiosity was piqued.

Most of the soymilk sold in the late 1980s was the powdered variety. I mixed it with water in half-gallon pitchers and stored it in my refrigerator. Aseptic cartons came later – they were convenient but expensive. Almond milk and rice milk were scarce, and most of the soymilk on the market wasn't fortified with calcium or vitamin D.

I enjoyed the mild, beany flavor of the soymilk and noticed an immediate change in my health. After I eliminated milk from my diet, I rarely caught a seasonal cold or flu again. Coincidence? Power of suggestion? Who knows, but the habit stuck.

Today, my diet is still largely dairy-free. I discovered in recent years that I'm allergic to soy foods and have replaced soymilk with fortified almond milk or rice milk. Luckily, finding these products is no longer a problem, because dairy alternatives have become mainstream. Who ever thought consumers would be buying almond milk at their neighborhood supermarkets? Not I, but I'm as pleased as can be.

Some cruise ship dining rooms also have table service and make food to order. In that case, you may be able to talk to wait staff about your needs and get some simple modifications to menu items to make them dairy-free.

If you have any concerns about whether the ship will be able to accommodate your special needs, ask in advance. Some cruise lines post their menus online so you can see the kinds of foods they serve ahead of time.

Planning for problems

Whether you've missed a flight and you and your dairy-free meal got separated or the restaurant at the hotel is closed, keep in mind that you can always make do. When you're traveling as a dairy-free eater, you have to be ready to improvise. Do your best to plan ahead, but be prepared to be flexible and find creative solutions when things don't go the way you'd hoped. And remember that your trip and the company you have are at the top of your priority list. Make it fun even if your meals aren't as great as you'd like them to be.

Stay positive, and think through your options. If you get desperate, try these tactics:

- **Eat what you can of the meal that was served.** If the flight attendant hands you the standard meal, pick the cheese off the sandwich and give the cheesecake to the guy sitting next to you.

- **Ask for extras.** When the flight attendants go around with the beverage service, ask for the full can of tomato juice or orange juice, and inquire about options for extra snack chips, cookies, or peanuts.

- **Buy what you can.** If you get stuck at a truck stop or convenience store when you're on the road, pick up the best of the worst. You'll survive. Now is the time to enjoy some popcorn and a bag of nuts or trail mix or to indulge in a bag of tortilla chips or box of graham crackers. Consider buying a small jar of peanut butter and a box of whole-grain crackers. They won't go to waste.

- **Pull out the reserves, if you brought them.** If you were able to bring along a sandwich from home, a carton of soymilk, and fresh fruit, now is the time to get it out.

There's no place like home. You'll always have your favorite, healthy, dairy-free foods available if you bring a little bit of home with you wherever you go. Make it a rule to travel with emergency supplies.

Chapter 17

Dairy-Free During Pregnancy and the Early Years

. . . .

In This Chapter

▶ Priming your body for pregnancy

▶ Understanding your nutritional needs

▶ Feeding your baby

▶ Taking care of toddlers

. . . .

When you're pregnant and later raising a baby, everyone gets more concerned about food. "You're eating for two now," is a figure of speech that highlights the fact that when you're pregnant, you're responsible for nourishing your own body as well as the baby developing inside you. After you give birth, you're responsible for ensuring that your child receives the proper nutrition. You want to make sure your children have a healthy start.

So what about the question of whether it's okay to start your child on a dairy-free diet? The answer: Of course it is. After all, people in many parts of the world have for thousands of years gone through pregnancies and raised young children without drinking milk from cows. You can, too.

In this chapter, I provide tips and advice for meeting your nutritional needs during a dairy-free pregnancy. And because your child's nutritional needs are just as important, I also explain how to move your baby from bottle or breast milk to dairy-free solids as well as how to ensure that her nutritional needs are met from baby to toddler.

Preparing for a Healthy, Dairy-Free Pregnancy

If you think you're possibly pregnant or if you're considering getting pregnant, eating a balanced diet is essential, especially if you're going dairy-free. Doing so ensures that your baby has the best possible start for a healthy life. The more time you have to prepare, the better. In this section, I explain how to get started.

I focus mostly on the dietary habits of pregnant women in this section, so if you have other pregnancy-related questions, check out *Pregnancy For Dummies,* 3rd Edition, by Joanne Stone, MD, Keith Eddleman, MD, and Mary Duenwald (Wiley).

Getting into nutritional shape before you get pregnant

No matter whether your pregnancy was planned or not, if you go into pregnancy well nourished, you and your baby can benefit from several health advantages. (If you're already pregnant but haven't been eating the best, don't waste any more time. Start now.) Ensuring that your body has all the vitamins, minerals, and other nutrients you need helps to support normal growth and development of the baby you're carrying. So anything you can do to be sure that you're eating well before getting pregnant is a good thing to do. After all, what you put into your body also goes into your baby's body. If you're well nourished, your baby will be well nourished.

Whether or not you eat dairy products, the advice for getting your diet in order before getting pregnant is basically the same for everybody. Here are the basics:

> ✔ **Follow your healthcare provider's advice about taking a multivitamin and mineral supplement for several months before you conceive.** In particular, current recommendations emphasize the importance of getting adequate *folic acid,* which is one of the B vitamins.
>
> Research has shown that getting plenty of folic acid before pregnancy may help protect your baby from having *neural tube defects,* such as spina bifida. *Spina bifida* is a type of birth defect that involves incomplete closure of the spinal cord.

✔ **Limit sweets such as candy, soft drinks, cakes, cookies, and pies as well as snack chips and other foods with little nutritional value.** Pregnancy is a time for maximizing the nutritional content of your diet, and junk foods displace foods that could be making a substantial contribution to the quality of your diet.

✔ **Control your caffeine intake.** If you drink coffee, limit it to no more than 2 to 3 cups a day. Similarly, limit your intake of caffeinated tea and soft drinks. The caffeine content of beverages varies, but 2 to 3 cups of coffee is roughly equal in caffeine content to about 5 cups of black tea or 6 cups of a cola soft drink.

✔ **Avoid alcoholic beverages and tobacco.** Steer clear of drinking alcohol or using tobacco if you think you have any chance of becoming pregnant, because you may be pregnant for several weeks before you know it. If you're using alcohol or tobacco during that time, you can harm your baby's health.

✔ **Drink plenty of water.** There's no hard-and-fast rule about the number of cups of water you need each day. However, pay attention to your level of thirst (especially in hot weather). Make it a habit to drink water often so you're always well hydrated. Fresh fruits and vegetables also are a good source of fluids.

✔ **Eat fresh fruits and vegetables regularly.** Fresh produce not only helps to keep you hydrated, but it also contains health-supporting phytochemicals not found in multivitamin and mineral supplements.

✔ **Get plenty of physical activity.** Exercise can help you maintain muscle tone and strength. It also promotes normal bowel movements at a time when many women experience constipation due to increased iron intake and a slowdown of the digestive system.

Take your healthcare provider's advice about the type and intensity of exercise you can engage in. However, walking usually is appropriate for most people.

✔ **Get enough sleep.** Being well rested supports health in many ways, including helping to keep your immune function strong. Most people need about eight hours of sleep per night.

Checking with a professional for tailored advice

All pregnant women need to take special care to eat well while they're expecting. Whether your diet includes dairy products or not, you still need to be aware of how pregnancy changes your dietary needs and how best to meet them. But, of course, those women with special diets must be extra vigilant.

If you have some special dietary needs but aren't sure how to deal with them, consider talking with your healthcare provider or a dietitian to get individualized dietary advice. Books such as this one are a good source of general information to give you some useful background and help you understand key issues. However, each woman has unique nutritional needs that may differ depending on her medical histories, biology, work and family considerations, and other factors.

So it's important to talk with a healthcare provider who's knowledgeable about your particular circumstances and can counsel you accordingly. For example, if you not only live dairy-free but also live as a vegetarian or vegan, you should make sure you get a reliable source of vitamin B12 in your diet. I talk more about vitamin B12 in Chapter 4.

Many women also start their pregnancies with low iron stores. If your iron stores aren't high enough when you begin your pregnancy, you may put yourself at risk for iron deficiency.

You may be surprised to learn that your blood volume increases by 50 percent during the course of your pregnancy. The extra fluid you carry dilutes your blood and can contribute to anemia if your iron stores aren't high enough at the outset. Your healthcare provider or dietician can help ensure that your iron stores are high enough.

Being dairy-free actually is an advantage where iron is concerned. That's because milk is low in iron. If you don't drink milk, you'll likely eat more foods rich in iron, such as cooked greens, beans, kale, cabbage, and broccoli.

Your healthcare provider can refer you to reliable resources about your prenatal care. Just be aware that many books and online materials may assume that you include dairy products in your diet, because that's the cultural norm in the United States. With the information I provide in this book, though, you should have the guidance you need to adapt the information in these sources to exclude dairy.

Obtaining the Nutrients Both of You Need

You're pregnant. Congratulations! Now that you have a bun in the oven, well-intentioned friends and family members may raise their eyebrows or wring their hands when they hear that you don't drink cow's milk. Pregnancy is a time when the people who love you hope everything works out well and that you have a healthy baby. So they may worry if your diet doesn't conform to the norm. No one has any reason to be concerned, though. You, as a human being, have no requirement for milk from a cow, and being pregnant doesn't change that.

To help you gather info to convince your family and friends of the safety of your diet, the following sections take a look at the dairy-free nutritional needs of you and your growing baby.

Choosing a prenatal supplement

If you didn't start taking a prenatal vitamin and mineral supplement before you were pregnant, your healthcare provider may recommend that you take one when you actually do become pregnant. That's standard advice for most pregnant women, whether or not they drink cow's milk.

Prenatal supplements don't take the place of a healthy diet, but they can fill any nutritional gaps you may have that may affect your growing baby. In particular, they're high in folic acid, iron, and calcium, nutrients that are especially important during pregnancy. When it comes to prenatal supplements, though, be sure to follow advice tailored for you as an individual by your doctor, dietitian, or other healthcare provider. (I include general information about supplements in Chapter 4.)

Taking a look at your nutrient needs

When you're pregnant, ensuring that you meet your nutrient needs is extra important because what you eat feeds the baby growing in your womb. If you don't consume good, nutritious foods, your baby won't receive what it needs to grow and develop properly. Dairy products do contain several important nutrients that your body needs. So, if you decide to pursue a dairy-free lifestyle, getting those nutrients from other sources is even more essential.

The good news: Your body was designed to get what you need during pregnancy without relying on a bovine beverage. If you're not consuming cow's milk, you want to ensure you're getting the most important nutrients found in the beverage: calcium, vitamin D, and vitamin B12. These nutrients are important to you while you're pregnant, so you want to pay particular attention to ensuring you get enough of them from other food sources. (In Chapter 4, I discuss these nutrients and dairy-free nutrition in more detail.)

In this section, I explain why calcium, vitamin D, and vitamin B12 are important and how to ensure that you get enough of these nutrients during your dairy-free pregnancy.

Sizing up your calcium needs

Pregnant women need about the same amount of calcium in their diets as they do when they're not pregnant. How much is that? About 1,000 milligrams per day. The figure stays the same when they're breastfeeding, too.

Still, whether they drink cow's milk or not, meeting recommended levels of calcium intake is a challenge for most women. When you're pregnant, however, it's important that you try. That's because calcium is an important component of bones and teeth for you and also your growing child.

Scientific evidence suggests that your body becomes more efficient at absorbing and retaining calcium during pregnancy, so you may have some built-in help to protect you and your baby if your calcium intake isn't quite up to recommended levels. Don't count on it, though. Your goal is to be as well nourished as possible before, during, and after pregnancy. It's best to aim for the 1,000 milligrams goal without relying on your body to work overtime.

If you need a little help boosting your calcium intake when you're pregnant, try these ideas:

- ✔ **Super-size your servings of calcium-rich foods.** Super-sizing doesn't just relate to burger and fry meals! Take double servings of cooked kale, broccoli, bok choy, baked beans, lentil soup, rice pudding (made with calcium-fortified soymilk), and other calcium-rich foods. (Check out Chapter 4 for more suggestions.)

- ✔ **Drink your calcium.** Drink 2 or 3 cups of calcium-fortified soymilk, rice milk, or almond milk each day or use it on your breakfast cereal. Drinking calcium-fortified fruit juices is an option, too (though fresh fruit is healthier because of the fiber it contains). Consider drinking up to ½ cup of juice daily.

  If you're having trouble getting all the calcium you need by drinking beverages, try cooking with it. You can use calcium-fortified nondairy milks to make cream soups. Check out the recipes I include in Chapter 10. You also can blend calcium-fortified soymilk, rice milk, or almond milk with fresh fruit and other wholesome ingredients to make smoothies. I include recipes in Chapter 14.

Watching your vitamin D intake

Vitamin D is a close partner to calcium — it helps your body absorb the calcium you take in. So, getting enough vitamin D during pregnancy helps ensure that you absorb that bone-building mineral. When you get the proper amount of both, your baby's bones and teeth develop normally.

Your primary nondairy sources of vitamin D when you're pregnant include your prenatal supplement, exposure to sunlight, and any vitamin D–fortified foods you may eat, including soymilk, rice milk, almond milk, orange juice, and breakfast cereals. Whole foods that contain vitamin D include eggs, tuna, salmon, and sardines. (Chapter 4 provides more information, including how much sunlight you need to get to produce the proper amount of vitamin D.)

Even though tuna and salmon contain vitamin D, they also may contain *mercury,* a neurotoxin that causes learning disabilities, lower IQs, and developmental delays in babies and children. Pregnant and nursing women, women in their childbearing years (ages 15 to 44), and all children and teens under the age of 15 are particularly vulnerable to this toxin. So this group of folks needs to be careful to avoid mercury-infused fish. If you decide to eat fish as a nondairy source of vitamin D, limit your intake. Eat no more than 5 ounces of canned tuna per week. Eat no more than one serving per month of Great Lakes salmon.

Mercury gets into fish through pollution from emissions from coal-fired power plants. Power plants spew mercury into the air, and then it falls into rivers and streams. Forests and wetlands also provide conditions that enhance the conversion of mercury into *methylmercury,* a highly toxic form that accumulates in fish.

For more information about potential hazards of eating fish when you're pregnant, check out the Environmental Protection Agency fish advisories Web site at `www.epa.gov/waterscience/fish`. Another good source of information is the nonprofit Environmental Working Group, which you can find at `www.ewg.org`.

Beefing up your vitamin B12 stores

Vitamin B12 is found only in animal products like meat, milk, fish, and poultry. If you don't eat any of these foods — because you're living dairy- and meat-free — be sure to include a reliable alternative source of vitamin B12 to your diet. You can get vitamin B12 from supplements and fortified foods. I provide more details and examples of good choices in Chapter 4.

Pregnant women need slightly more vitamin B12 when they're pregnant as compared to before they became pregnant. It's critically important to get enough vitamin B12 during pregnancy and when you're breastfeeding. Vitamin B12 is needed for proper development of the baby's brain and nervous system. Getting enough vitamin B12 also helps ensure normal formation of red blood cells.

Hello Baby! Welcoming Your Newest Dairy-Free Family Member

Welcome to a world in which the inhabitants wear mashed potatoes in their hair and stick peas in their ears. Your entry into the realm of feeding a baby is bound to be an adventure. If you're planning to launch your child on a dairy-free diet, the information I include in this section will be indispensible.

Feeding any child takes time and care, so you want to be fully informed. This way you can feed your child a healthful diet with confidence. You also want to be prepared to answer questions from curious family members and friends who may be unfamiliar with the facts and feel worried or concerned about your child's diet because it's different from the way of eating they've always known.

In this section, I cover important information about options for feeding your baby throughout her first year. I include information about milk allergies and baby formulas as well as detailed instructions for making the transition from breast or bottle to dairy-free solid foods.

Breast or bottle: Looking at your feeding choices

Nobody is born ready to eat a cheeseburger. Humans all enter this world and drink milk at first. They ease into their diets over a period of a few years. From the start, all that babies can tolerate is an easy-to-digest slurry of fluids filled with vital nutrients and other substances. These ingredients promote the rapid growth and development that happens immediately after birth.

The most natural source of this nourishment is mother's milk or a close replica (such as formula). Milk in some form is a baby's food for the first four to six months of life. Babies need no other source of calories during this time.

In fact, babies who are given solid foods too soon are at greater risk of becoming overweight or developing food allergies. Those solid foods also may displace vital nutrients needed from breast milk or baby formula. Resist the temptation to give solids to babies younger than 4 to 6 months of age.

Either of the following choices — breastfeeding or bottlefeeding — may be an option for you and your baby, depending on your circumstances. It's important to understand the rationale for each and make the decision that's best for you.

Breastfeeding: Mother's milk is best

Without a doubt, the very best food for babies through the first six months of life (and longer, if possible) is breast milk. Breast milk holds advantages over other options for several reasons. They include the following:

- ✔ **The composition of breast milk is optimal.** Because milk is species-specific, human milk naturally contains the precise mix of nutrients — proteins, fats, carbohydrates, vitamins, and minerals — needed for a human baby's growth and development.

  Even well-designed substitutes — commercial baby formulas — aren't likely to be as good as breast milk. Scientists are in the process of discovering that substances in whole foods that are important for human health aren't available in supplements. Similarly, breast milk may contain health-supporting substances that aren't already identified and included in synthetic formulas.

- ✔ **It contains immunity boosters.** Substances present in human breast milk strengthen a baby's immune system and give him added protection against certain illnesses. Breastfed babies also are less likely to develop allergies later in life.

- ✔ **Breastfeeding promotes ideal weight.** Babies who are breastfed are less likely to be overweight or obese later in life.

- ✔ **It's convenient and sterile.** Breast milk is always ready and at the right temperature. It's also sterile when it comes directly from Mom, so it's free of bacteria that maybe lurking in unclean bottles or formula that's been sitting out too long.

- ✔ **Breastfeeding helps Mom get back into shape.** When you breastfeed an infant, it causes your uterus to contract, helping it return to its pre-pregnancy condition. Also, when you're breastfeeding, you need about 200 calories a day more than when you were pregnant. That means that women who are breastfeeding need about 500 calories per day more than they ate before they got pregnant. The fact that you need so many extra calories when you're breastfeeding is why breastfeeding is such a good idea. Not only does it nourish your baby with the best food possible, but it can also help a woman take off extra pounds gained during the pregnancy.

It's ideal when women breastfeed their babies, but for a number of reasons it may not be possible for some women. So, it's important not to chastise or make women who don't breastfeed feel badly about their choice.

Going over some bottle basics

Breastfeeding sometimes can be difficult or impossible for a woman. The reasons are varied and may include health issues related to the baby or the mom. Or a mom may have a problem with her breast milk itself — it may contain environmental contaminants or other undesirable substances that may be transmitted through the milk.

Luckily, when you can't breastfeed, you do have an alternative: synthetic infant formula. Several brands of infant formula are available on the market. Your healthcare provider can recommend a few to you. In most cases, you can buy these at supermarkets, discount stores, or even some warehouse stores.

Most infant formulas are based on cow's milk, which is altered to be more easily digested and to more closely resemble human breast milk. Infant formulas that are made with cow's milk are identified as "milk-based" on the front label of the products. If you want your baby to avoid cow's milk, don't use these products. In this case, other infant formulas that contain no animal products are available. Most of these are soy-based products. Typical brands include Isomil and Prosobee.

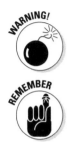

Commercial soymilk meant for general use (such as Silk, Organic Valley, and EdenSoy) isn't the same thing as infant soy formula. Soymilk is fine for older children, but it isn't appropriate for infants and young toddlers.

If your baby is bottle fed, don't put anything in the bottle except breast milk, formula, or water for the first six months. Sugar-water drinks, soft drinks, and iced tea are inappropriate for babies and small children. Fruit juices and diluted baby cereals shouldn't be introduced until after the six-month point. When these products are introduced, they should be given in a cup or by spoon, not in a bottle, to discourage the formation of cavities in baby teeth. Nothing is more nutritious or beneficial to your baby for the first six months than breast milk or commercial infant formula. Talk to your healthcare provider to find out whether your baby needs water to supplement the milk or formula she's getting.

Identifying infant milk allergies

Some babies have to avoid milk-based infant formulas because they're allergic to cow's milk. Specifically, they're allergic to one of the proteins in cow's milk. Casein is one example of a milk protein found in milk-based infant formulas as well as in many processed foods. I include examples of those foods in Chapter 5. I also explain milk allergies in much more detail in Chapter 2.

Babies with a milk allergy may be excessively fussy and irritable. They may have other symptoms, too, including diarrhea or loose, bloody stools. Your healthcare provider can run tests to diagnose a milk allergy.

Testing for a milk allergy involves the following options:

✔ **Blood tests:** A sample of blood is taken from your child and checked for antibodies that suggest a sensitivity to milk protein. *Antibodies,* or immunoglobulins, are proteins produced by the body to fight foreign substances, such as bacteria or viruses, when they're present in your system.

If your child is allergic to a cow's milk protein, his body may produce antibodies when the milk protein is present. Babies who are allergic to cow's milk sometimes also are allergic to the protein in soy-based formulas.

✔ **Skin tests:** Your child's skin is scratched and exposed to a milk protein. If your child is allergic to the protein, the area that was exposed to the allergen will react with a *hive,* or raised, red bump.

Neither of these tests is foolproof, but both can help your healthcare provider hone in on the most likely explanation for your child's symptoms. A milk allergy in children usually occurs in the early years up to about age 3. After that, the allergy usually begins to go away.

Supplementing your baby's diet with dairy-free solids

Between 4 and 6 months of age, your child may show signs of being ready to include some solids in her diet. For instance, when your baby is able to sit up independently and grab for things to put into her mouth, it's time to begin introducing solid foods.

You won't find hard-and-fast rules about how to introduce solid foods to babies. Instead, you can follow some general guidelines. For example, all babies — whether they're dairy-free or not — start out eating foods that are easy for immature digestive systems to handle. They also start with foods that are the least likely to cause problems, such as allergic reactions or choking.

Foods that are easiest to tolerate include nondairy cooked cereals initially and later mashed or puréed fruits and vegetables and their juices. Baby rice cereal is the most common first food, because rice is hypoallergenic. Most babies tolerate it well. (It's best to feed your baby iron-fortified baby rice cereal until she's at least 18 months old.) Other fortified baby cereals, including oat and wheat cereals, also can be used.

The best way to introduce solids is to start with small amounts of foods, one at a time. Begin gradually, alternating with breast or bottle feedings. You can mix baby rice cereal with breast milk or infant formula and offer a few tablespoons. Work up to two feedings a day, totaling about ½ cup. From there, you'll gradually add other foods, one at a time, a little at a time. Your baby will increase the amounts at her own pace. By introducing new foods one at a time, it's easier to pinpoint troublesome foods if your baby shows signs of food sensitivity.

You should wait until your baby is older before introducing protein-rich foods and foods that are high in fat. Foods such as meats, nut butters, and even non-dairy cheeses are more difficult for immature digestive systems to manage. After your baby has adjusted to cooked cereals and mashed and puréed fruits and vegetables, you can move to nondairy table foods.

Even in families that aren't living dairy-free, fluid cow's milk is off-limits for infants under the age of one year. That's because drinking cows' milk can cause bleeding in the gastrointestinal tract and lead to anemia. Infants given cow's milk also have been shown in some studies to have an increased risk for insulin-dependent diabetes. (Trace amounts of dairy products in other foods aren't as likely to cause a problem.)

Introducing dairy-free food during the first year

Solids are introduced slowly, a few foods at a time, starting at around 4 to 6 months of age (see the preceding section). The rules aren't carved into stone for how to progress, but Table 17-1 provides a reasonable schedule for feeding dairy-free babies from 4 through 12 months of age.

Taking note of other important pieces of nutritional advice for your baby

Keep in mind a few other nutritional pointers for your baby's diet during the first year. They include the following:

✔ If you're living dairy-free and also eat no other animal products (you're a vegan), it's critical that you take a vitamin B12 supplement while you're breastfeeding. Doing so ensures that your baby has a source of vitamin B12.

✔ If you have concerns about whether your baby is getting enough vitamin D, check

in with your healthcare provider. The current recommendation is to start a vitamin D supplement of 400 IU shortly after birth for breastfed infants.

✔ Babies who are breastfed usually are started on iron supplements when they turn 4 to 6 months of age. You should check in with your healthcare provider for more information.

Table 17-1	Feeding Dairy-Free Babies Ages 4 to 12 Months			
	4 to 7 Months	*6 to 8 Months*	*7 to 10 Months*	*10 to 12 Months*
Milk	Breast milk or soy formula	Breast milk or soy formula	Breast milk or soy formula	Breast milk or soy formula (24 to 32 ounces)
Cereal & Bread	Begin iron-fortified baby cereal mixed with breast milk or formula	Continue baby cereal; begin other breads and cereals	Continue baby cereal and other breads and cereals	Continue baby cereal and breads until 18 months; feed a total of 4 servings (1 serving = ¼ slice bread or 2 to 4 tablespoons cereal)
Fruits & Vegetables	None	Begin juice from cup (2 to 4 ounces of a vitamin C source); begin mashed vegetables and fruits	Continue with 4 ounces juice; add pieces of soft/cooked fruits and vegetables	Begin a table-food diet; allow 4 servings per day (1 serving = 2 to 4 table-spoons fruits and vegetables and 4 ounces of juice)
Protein-Rich Foods	None	None	Gradually introduce tofu, casseroles, puréed legumes, puréed meats (meatless diets are healthier, however), nondairy cheese, and soy yogurt	Provide 2 servings of protein daily, each about ½ ounce; nut butters shouldn't be started before 1 year of age

Note: Overlap of age ranges occurs due to varying rates of development. Adapted from Simply Vegan: Quick Vegetarian Meals, 4th Edition, by Debra Wasserman and Reed Mangels, PhD, RD, 2006. Reprinted with permission from The Vegetarian Resource Group, P.O. Box 1463, Baltimore, MD 21203; phone 410-366-8343; Web site www.vrg.org.

As Your Child Ages: Feeding during the Twos and Threes

Establishing healthful eating habits in childhood is more important than at any other time in life. That's because the habits your child forms early on in life are likely to follow him into adulthood and influence his long-term health.

You have nearly total control over your child's diet when he's an infant. However, as soon as he begins eating solid foods, he'll have opportunities to express food preferences and even make some food choices of his own.

 If you want to feed your toddler a diet that's free of dairy products, doing so is okay. You can ensure he's well nourished without milk products. As I discuss in Part I of this book, no human nutritional needs require you or your children to drink milk from a cow.

Sometimes the more immediate concerns for your toddler are related to issues that all parents face, regardless of whether their child eats dairy products. I show you how to plan some dairy-free meals and snacks in the following sections. Understanding how to prepare wholesome meals and snacks will make your toddler's dairy-free diet much easier to manage.

Planning meals without dairy

The key to planning healthful, dairy-free meals for your toddler is to include a wide variety of wholesome foods. Encouraging your child to try a variety of new tastes and textures also is a good idea.

Dealing with food jags

Toddlers are notorious for their food jags. *Food jags* are basically the sporadic food preferences younger children have. For example, this week your children may love carrots, and then next week they may really hate them. A 3-year-old can eat nothing but graham crackers for days before deciding that applesauce is her favorite food.

Such strong food preferences are typical of children this age. They can last for weeks or even months. Your best strategy for dealing with food jags is to take them in stride and to not overreact. You have no reason to worry about these fickle food preferences. Fortunately, they're usually short-lived and aren't likely to do any harm. Toddlers soon outgrow them and begin to eat more consistently.

The greater the range of foods your child learns to like, the more likely it is that she'll get all the nutrients she needs. Table 17-2 shows a daily, dairy-free feeding guide for toddlers and preschoolers ages 1 to 3.

Table 17-2	Meal Planning Guide for Toddlers and Preschoolers Ages 1 to 3	
Food Group	_Number of Servings_	_Example of One Serving_
Grains	6 or more	½ to 1 slice bread; ¼ to ½ cup cooked cereal, grain, or pasta; ½ to ¾ cup ready-to-eat cereal
Protein-rich foods	2 or more	¼ to ½ cup cooked beans, tofu, tempeh, or textured vegetable protein; 1½ to 3 ounces lean meat
Fortified soymilk and so on	3	1 cup fortified soymilk, infant formula, or breast milk
Vegetables	2 or more	¼ to ½ cup cooked vegetables or ½ to 1 cup raw vegetables
Fruits	3 or more	¼ to ½ cup canned fruit; ½ cup juice; 1 medium-sized piece of fruit
Fats	3	1 teaspoon trans-fat-free margarine or oil; use ½ teaspoon flaxseed oil or 2 teaspoons canola oil daily to supply omega-3 fatty acids

Adapted from Simply Vegan: Quick Vegetarian Meals, 4th Edition, by Debra Wasserman and Reed Mangels, PhD, RD, 2006. Reprinted with permission from The Vegetarian Resource Group, P.O. Box 1463, Baltimore, MD 21203; phone 410-366-8343; Web site www.vrg.org.

Raising vegan children

Some families go all the way and not only exclude dairy products from their diets but also meat, fish, poultry, and eggs, too. They opt for a _vegan diet,_ which is free of all animal products and byproducts (including honey!). Young children can thrive on diets that exclude all animal products. If you decide to raise a vegan child, check out my book, _Living Vegetarian For Dummies_ (Wiley) for all the details.

Children who eat a vegan diet need slightly more protein than other children because of the differences in the digestibility and composition of plant and animal proteins. Still, if vegan children get enough calories to meet their energy needs and eat a reasonable variety of foods, they can get plenty of protein in their diets.

You do need to make sure, however, that your vegan child has a reliable source of vitamin B12 in her diet. I list examples in Chapter 4. If your child has limited exposure to sunshine, she also may need a vitamin D supplement. Check with your healthcare provider for an individualized assessment and advice.

Making sensible dairy-free snacks

Young children need frequent opportunities to eat. That's because the healthiest dairy-free foods — fresh fruits and vegetables, whole grains, and legumes — are bulky. Young children have small stomachs and fill up on these foods quickly. Between-meal snacks offer the extra calories they need to meet their energy needs.

The most healthful dairy-free snacks are low in sodium, saturated fat, trans fat, and added sugar. They're high in fiber, too. Examples of good choices include

- ✔ Cooked or dry cereal with fortified soymilk, almond milk, or rice milk
- ✔ Cut up veggies with nondairy dip or hummus
- ✔ Fresh fruit cut into kid-friendly pieces
- ✔ Homemade whole-grain mini muffins
- ✔ Pudding made with fortified nondairy milk
- ✔ Soy yogurt
- ✔ Unsweetened applesauce with a sprinkle of cinnamon

Relying on dairy-free vegetarian options

Looking for some quick and convenient dairy-free snack or meal ideas? Try the vegetarian options at your local natural foods store. Most vegetarian entrees and snack items labeled as being suitable for vegetarians actually are vegan. That means they're dairy-free. Yeah! (See the nearby sidebar "Raising vegan children" for more information.)

Examples include many frozen foods, such as burritos, ethnic entrees, vegetarian pizzas, rice bowls, and other meals. It's worth a trip to your local natural foods store to see what you may find that may appeal to a picky toddler or older child.

Resources for learning more

Some of the best sources of information and recipes for dairy-free living come from vegetarian literature, especially cookbooks and Web sites. Even if you don't care to go vegetarian, you can get lots of ideas and good information about living dairy-free from these sources. I list a few of my favorite books here:

- *Vegan Lunch Box: 130 Amazing, Animal-Free Lunches Kids and Grown-Ups Will Love!* by Jennifer McCann (Da Capo Press)

- *Healthy Eating for Life for Children* by the Physicians Committee for Responsible Medicine with Amy Lanou (Wiley)

- *The Ultimate Uncheese Cookbook: Delicious Dairy-Free Cheeses and Classic "Uncheese" Dishes,* 10th Anniversary Edition, by Joanne Stepaniak (Book Publishing Company)

- *The Vegetarian Family Cookbook* by Nava Atlas (Broadway)

- *Simply Vegan: Quick Vegetarian Meals,* 4th Edition, by Debra Wasserman and Reed Mangels, PhD, RD (Vegetarian Resource Group)

You also can visit the Vegetarian Resource Group Web site at www.vrg.org. The Vegetarian Resource Group (VRG) is a U.S. nonprofit organization that educates the public about the interrelated issues of health, nutrition, ecology, ethics, and world hunger. The group publishes the bimonthly *Vegetarian Journal* and provides numerous other printed materials for consumers and health professionals. Materials are provided free of charge or at a modest cost in bulk, and many are available in Spanish. The VRG health and nutrition materials are peer reviewed by registered dietitians and physicians.

Chapter 18

Raising Happy, Healthy Dairy-Free Kids and Teens

*F*or the most part, kids aren't too difficult to please. Although some of them may be picky eaters, generally they just want foods that taste good and are easy to eat. You don't have to serve them anything fancy. If foods are colorful, easy to scoop with a spoon or fork, or can be eaten with their fingers, they're happy.

When you raise kids on a dairy-free diet, getting them to eat certain foods isn't that much different than on a regular diet. All you have to do is accentuate the positive and show them all the good-tasting, nondairy options they have. And there are plenty of them.

You can make most of the decisions when your child is young, but eventually he'll be on his own. So be sure to use the time that your children are with you to instill strong values about food and nutrition. Help them gain the knowledge and skills through hands-on experiences with growing, planning, preparing, and eating healthful, dairy-free meals. By teaching your children how to live dairy-free today, you can equip them with the skills they'll take into adulthood.

In this chapter, I show you how to provide your kids with a nutritious, nondairy diet that gives them what they need for optimal growth and development. I cover meal management at home and how to work through certain challenges, such as dealing with meals at school, parties, and other social events where food may take center stage. I also discuss ways to empower your kids to take charge of their own diets and make their own good food choices.

Making Sure Dairy-Free Kids Grow Up Healthy and Happy

Dairy products are a mainstay in the diets of many children. Just look at the kids' menu at your favorite family restaurant. You see the usual line-up: macaroni and cheese, grilled cheese sandwiches, pizza, and ice cream. Similar foods are favorites at their friends' parties, too. You also can't forget that carton of milk with the school lunch and that glass of milk with cookies later on at home.

You can clearly see that today's society has a strong tradition of including lots of dairy products in kids' diets. But despite the fact that children eat large amounts of dairy, no scientific rationale exists for serving it. Sure, kids need nutrients found in cow's milk, but cow's milk isn't the only food source of those nutrients. Many other foods are rich sources of calcium and vitamin D, too. Just as good nondairy sources of calcium are available for adults, many alternatives — most of which are more healthful than cow's milk — are available for kids, too. It's all a matter of making them available and appealing to children.

In the following sections, I focus on dairy-free nutrition for kids, including what they need and how they can build strong bones and teeth without consuming cow's milk. I help you get your head around what you need to know and put it all into perspective.

Understanding their nutritional needs

Feeding children takes time, patience, and care no matter whether they eat dairy products or not. Any diet that doesn't take basic principles of nutrition into consideration or that is planned haphazardly risks being inadequate. So, if your child's diet is heavy on French fries and soft drinks and light on fruits and vegetables, it's not likely to give your kids what they need to thrive — whether they're dairy-free or not.

If you desire (or need) to go dairy-free with your children's diet, the good news is that doing so isn't overly difficult. A healthful, dairy-free diet includes plenty of fresh fruits and vegetables, whole-grain breads and cereals, beans and peas, and seeds and nuts. Whenever possible, these foods should be as close to their natural state as possible instead of highly processed. In other words, it's your job to teach your kids to eat the potato, not the potato chip.

In Table 18-1, I provide a meal-planning guide for children from 4 to 13 years of age. This guide excludes all dairy products. In place of these dairy products are fortified substitutes such as soymilk and lots of beans and greens. These foods are concentrated sources of calcium and other nutrients that are vital to the growth and development of young bodies.

Table 18-1	Meal-Planning Guide for Children Ages 4 to 13	
Food Group	**Number of Servings**	**Example of One Serving**
Grains	8 or more for 4- to 8-year-olds; 10 or more for 9- to 13-year-olds	1 slice of bread; ½ cup cooked cereal, grain, or pasta; ¾ cup ready-to-eat cereal
Protein foods	5 or more for 4- to 8-year-olds; 6 or more for 9- to 13-year-olds	½ cup cooked beans, tofu*, tempeh, or textured vegetable protein; 1 cup fortified soymilk*; 1 ounce of lean meat or meat substitute; ¼ cup nuts or seeds*; 2 tablespoons nut or seed butter*
Vegetables	4 or more	½ cup cooked or 1 cup raw vegetables*
Fruits	2 or more	½ cup canned fruit; ½ cup fruit juice; 1 medium piece of fruit
Fats	2 or more for 4- to 8-year-olds; 3 or more for 9- to 13-year-olds	1 teaspoon trans-fat-free margarine or oil
Omega-3 Fats	1 per day	1 teaspoon flaxseed oil; 1 tablespoon canola or soybean oil; 1 tablespoon ground flaxseed; ¼ cup walnuts

* Starred Food Items: 6 or more servings for 4- to 8-year-olds; 10 or more for 9- to 13-year-olds (1 serving = ½ cup calcium-set tofu; 1 cup calcium-fortified soymilk, orange juice, or soy yogurt; ¼ cup almonds; 2 tablespoons tahini or almond butter; 1 cup cooked or 2 cups raw broccoli, bok choy, collards, kale, or mustard greens). These also count as servings from the other groups at the same time. They aren't additional. These are the foods you want because they are high in calcium.

Notes: The calorie content of the diet can be increased by greater amounts of nut butters, dried fruits, soy products, and other high-calorie foods. Children who are vegetarian and eat no animal products at all should regularly consume a source of vitamin B12 like Vegetarian Support Formula nutritional yeast, vitamin B12–fortified soymilk, vitamin B12–fortified breakfast cereal, vitamin B12–fortified meat substitute, or vitamin B12 supplements. Adequate exposure to sunlight — 20 to 30 minutes of summer sun on hands and face two to three times a week — is recommended to promote vitamin D synthesis. If sunlight exposure is limited, supplemental vitamin D should be used.

Adapted from Simply Vegan: Quick Vegetarian Meals, 4th Edition, by Debra Wasserman and Reed Mangels, PhD, RD. Adapted with permission from The Vegetarian Resource Group, P.O. Box 1463, Baltimore, MD 21203; phone 410-366-8343; Web site www.vrg.org.

A good way to help judge whether your child is getting what he needs is to plot his growth on a growth chart. You can find and download these charts online or get them from your pediatrician. Use a growth chart to follow your child's height and weight at regular intervals and compare them to population norms. Growth rates are reported in percentiles, and they may vary from child to child. For example, my child may be growing at the 50th percentile for height and weight, and yours may be at the 90th percentile. One growth rate isn't necessarily better or healthier than another. What's most important is that your child grows at a consistent rate and doesn't falter.

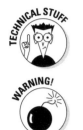

Within populations, it's expected that half of the people are growing at the 50th percentile, one-quarter are growing at the 25th percentile, and so on. Scientists call this *normal distribution.*

The time to worry about your child's growth rate is if you notice a drastic fall-off in his rate of growth. For example, if your child was growing at the 50th percentile and suddenly fell to a growth rate at the 25th percentile, you would want to determine the reason for the change. Your child's healthcare provider will investigate a drop in the rate of growth such as this, so make an appointment with her.

Another good way to ensure that your child gets what he needs is to encourage him to eat a variety of healthful foods and to minimize foods with little nutritional value. He also needs to get enough calories to meet his energy needs and help him grow at a steady rate. I include a list of healthful, dairy-free snacks later in this chapter.

Building healthy bones and teeth

What's the issue of most concern to parents when they think about a non-dairy diet for their kids? Teeth and bones! They want to be sure their children grow up with healthy ones. To get strong teeth and bones, kids need the proper amount of calcium and vitamin D. In the following sections, I dig in to these topics in detail.

Keeping an eye on calcium

Children's and teens' bodies are in a phase of rapid growth and development. As a result, they need plenty of *calcium,* a mineral that's important for the proper development of their teeth and bones. So, it's only natural to wonder where they'll get the calcium they need if they don't drink milk or eat other dairy products.

Here's the good news: Your child can get enough calcium on a dairy-free diet, but like any healthful diet, it takes care and planning. It also takes dedication to a wholesome diet limited in the *junk foods* — candies, chips, and other empty-calorie foods — that can squeeze healthier foods out of the diet.

The Food and Nutrition Board of the Institute of Medicine of the National Academies recommends that children and teens age 9 through 18 get 1,300 milligrams of calcium every day. Younger children ages 4 through 8 need less — about 800 milligrams every day — and children ages 1 through 3 need about 500 milligrams. That's a lot of calcium for children in each of those age categories to eat, but other factors are just as important as the actual amount of calcium in the diet. The presence of vitamin D as well as factors that affect the absorption and retention of calcium by the body make a big difference. I discuss these absorption and retention factors in detail in Chapter 4. And you can read more about vitamin D in the following section.

To ensure that your child gets enough calcium, encourage her to eat four good-sized servings of calcium-rich foods every day. You don't need to be precise about how big the serving is. About a half cup of cooked vegetables (or one cup if raw) per serving is enough; more is even better. (Cooked vegetables are more compact than raw, so cooked vegetables generally contain a greater concentration of minerals and some vitamins as compared to raw.)

I list good sources of calcium in Chapter 4, but some that are particularly well liked by kids include the following:

- **Broccoli:** Broccoli has a fun shape, good flavor, and a texture kids like. Break up raw broccoli into florets and let kids dip them into dairy-free salad dressings or hummus. Or stand broccoli stalks up in a pan and steam them, serving them like a little broccoli forest with a dab of non-dairy margarine melted on top.

- **Calcium-fortified orange juice:** Nutritionists now recommend that kids drink no more than a half cup of fruit juice each day. That's because caloric drinks promote obesity, a major public health problem today. If your child drinks juice, choose fortified varieties. You also can freeze fortified orange juice in ice cube trays or molds to make frozen treats.

- **Calcium-fortified soymilk:** Vanilla and chocolate flavors of soymilk are favorites among children and teens. Besides just serving them for breakfast and dinner and with cookies, try using them to make smoothies and nondairy ice cream. I include recipes for both in Chapter 14.

- **Refried beans:** Refried beans (made without added lard) are rich in fiber, vitamins, and minerals in addition to calcium. Use them to make burritos, nachos, and tacos. For a fun and easy lunch or dinner, set up a burrito or taco bar in your kitchen, setting out toppings such as chopped lettuce and tomatoes, shredded nondairy cheese, salsa, chopped broccoli, and of course beans! For an alternative to store-bought refried beans, mash your own cooked black beans or pinto beans.

Shining a light on vitamin D

Vitamin D is the other nutrient that bears special attention where kids are concerned. *Vitamin D* is a hormone that works in tandem with calcium to produce strong bones and teeth. You can read more about this relationship in Chapter 4. Though kids can get vitamin D through fortified soymilk, rice milk, and almond milk, exposure to sunlight is their primary source. I discuss sunlight exposure — how much and for how long — in Chapter 4.

The Food and Nutrition Board of the Institute of Medicine of the National Academies recommends 5 micrograms (200 IUs) of cholecalciferol, a form of vitamin D, for boys and girls from birth through adulthood (up to age 50) if they don't get what they need from sunlight exposure. Scientists currently are considering a recommendation to increase this amount as well.

If you have concerns about whether your child may be getting the vitamin D he needs, check in with a registered dietitian or your healthcare provider. She can do an assessment of your child and make any necessary recommendations.

Thinking through the decision to raise dairy-free kids

If you plan to raise your child on a dairy-free diet, it's wise to give some thought to the challenges you may face in helping her avoid the foods that you don't want her to have (or that she can't have due to health-related issues) while also ensuring that she gets the nutrition she needs. Going dairy-free isn't a trivial matter.

Eating a diet that's outside the norm among her friends may require you to teach your child some coping skills and lessons she can apply when she has to make her own decisions about what to eat (and not eat). After all, you won't always be there to make the choice for her. I go into more detail about some of these situations — and offer some advice — later in this chapter.

If you decide to go dairy-free with your kids, you may need some training as well, because building meals that don't include dairy may be outside your skill set, too. This book is a great start, but you need practice before you become an expert. While you're in the learning phase, monitoring and supporting your child's diet require extra time and attention. I provide some targeted tips and advice later in this chapter.

Helping children learn about good nutrition and supporting them in eating healthful meals are important and challenging jobs for parents. These jobs are an even greater challenge if your child is on a special diet that's different from his peers'. So know going into this decision that you're adding a layer of complexity to the job by going dairy-free. Going dairy-free is a healthy choice, of course, but it helps to be aware of the challenges so you can adjust your expectations accordingly.

Preparing for doubters

One expectation you may need to adjust — or at least prepare for — pertains to people giving you unsolicited advice about your child's diet. Friends and family members may mean well when they express concerns about your child's diet. They have the same questions you may have had before you were educated about the issues. Some people are less inclined to part with tradition, too, and they may feel that by avoiding dairy products, you're somehow rejecting their values or their love.

 Use your own judgment if you find yourself in this situation. From my experience, the best response to someone who questions your approach to your child's diet is to politely listen, thank the person for the input, think about whether you'd like to follow up on the advice, and then quietly return to your own business.

The best way to equip yourself to stand up to long-standing food traditions is knowledge. Educate yourself about the nutrition facts of a dairy-free diet so you can be confident about your choices and those you make for your family.

Making Sure Your Kids Are On Board with Their Meals

As anyone with kids can tell you, you can't force someone to eat something she doesn't want to. If you try, you'll later find those foods hidden under knives, plate edges, or napkins. You may find a few peas in pockets, too. Convincing kids that the foods that are good for them also are tasty to eat is much easier than enduring a dinnertime dictatorship. You can use some strategies to help achieve this goal of getting them on board.

In this section, I share a few ideas for getting your child interested in your healthful meals and making her think that eating those foods was her idea.

Getting them involved

Here's a news flash you should know about: Kids are more likely to eat meals that they've had a hand in planning and preparing. So the more you can involve your child in the process of meal planning and preparation, the more interested he'll be in the meal. And the more interested he is, the more likely he'll be to actually eat the food you serve.

You have several ways to get Junior involved. Here are some ideas:

- ✔ **Take your child shopping.** If you're picking out apples, let him choose. Don't worry about whether he picks the best ones. Just let him have the experience of participating and helping. Older children can be given more responsibility. Give the child a short list or an item or two to locate on the other side of the store. Let him choose among the heads of lettuce or cartons of soymilk and bring them back to the cart.

- ✔ **Involve your child in meal planning.** Talk about the menu for the meal together and let him offer suggestions or make some simple choices among side dishes. As the parent, you need to coach your child to choose healthy foods — not chicken nuggets and macaroni and cheese every night.

- ✔ **Let the kids cook.** Supervise young children but let them help with simple tasks such as bringing items to you from the pantry, dumping ingredients into a pot or bowl, or shucking corn. Older children can help with such tasks as peeling fruits and vegetables with a paring knife or peeler, stirring pots on the stove, or assembling items for casseroles, soups, or other dishes.

- ✔ **Expect your child to help with other tasks.** Setting and clearing the table are ways he can contribute to the family meal. Loading and emptying the dishwasher — or helping to wash dishes by hand — are other meal-related tasks kids can help manage.

- ✔ **Grow your own ingredients.** Planning, planting, and tending a garden are great ways to teach your child about how food grows. Successful gardening also encourages an appreciation for fresh foods, gives your child a sense of accomplishment, and bolsters his self-esteem.

If you don't have space for a full-sized garden or don't have the time to tend one, downsize your ideas. Plant a windowsill herb garden, or grow tomatoes and peppers in pots in your backyard. For inspiration, check out *Vegetable Gardening For Dummies,* 2nd Edition, by Charlie Nardozzi (Wiley).

Modeling healthy choices

It may sound simple, but one of the best ways to get your kids to embrace a dairy-free lifestyle is simple. Model the behavior you want your children to emulate. Your kids notice what you eat, and they notice when you don't eat your vegetables, too. Be a role model and demonstrate that you enjoy and indulge in tasty foods that are good for you. For example, if you would like your kids to eat broccoli and whole-grain cereals with fortified almond milk, let them see you eating those foods, too.

Present healthful foods with a positive attitude, too. Project the expectation that you love the foods you're fixing and that you anticipate your kids will like them, too.

Don't pretend to like something you don't. Kids can spot a faker. If you don't care for a particular food that you'd like your kids to try — soymilk, rice milk, or a whole-wheat bagel with nondairy cream cheese — serve it to your kids but don't play up the fact that you aren't joining in.

Giving them a voice

Everyone wants a choice. Kids are no exception. In fact, having the experience of making their own choices, including decisions about what to eat, is an important aspect of children's emotional growth and development.

Mealtime is one of those opportunities to let your kids flex their decision-making muscles. If they have a choice, they're less likely to reject a food outright. For example, instead of telling your child to use soymilk on cereal, you may offer a choice of vanilla-flavored soymilk or plain rice milk to put on her morning cereal.

For very young children, you may want to offer a limited range of choices to help ensure that they stay within certain food parameters and get what they need nutritionally. For dessert, for example, you can offer applesauce or pear slices. For their sandwich, ask whether they'd like a whole-grain pita pocket or slices of whole-wheat bread.

Older children may be able to handle a wider range of choices, and they may express some special requests, too. It's okay to entertain special requests within reason, especially if it encourages your child to get involved with meal planning. For example, your child may suggest that you fix a burrito bar for dinner, or maybe she's in the mood for homemade mac and cheese made with nondairy cheese and plain soymilk.

Working through the Challenges

Living dairy-free may present you with some food situations with regard to your children that are new to you. Even though the learning curve is steep, in time, managing these challenges will become second nature to you. Until they do, this section provides some pointers for dealing with the challenges as effectively as possible.

Handling picky eaters

Children have food preferences just like you and me. Some of their preferences change over time as they mature and are exposed to a greater variety of flavors, textures, and aromas. In the meantime, they may hate carrots today and love them next week. They may like the consistency of mashed potatoes and dislike the skin on a baked potato.

If you're raising a picky eater, try these strategies to encourage him to experiment with a wide range of nondairy alternatives:

- ✔ **Give him a choice.** As I mention earlier in the chapter, giving kids a choice between foods helps get them interested in the meal and counteracts resistance to specific foods. Even picky eaters are likely to respond to having options. For example, if your child turns up his nose at a dish of soy yogurt, offer him a choice of nondairy rice pudding instead.

- ✔ **Don't push.** If you offer choices but your child still doesn't want to eat the foods you've offered, let it go. Attempting to force or cajole your child into eating something he's decided he doesn't want is likely to produce a power struggle you can't win. Instead, wait until the next meal or snack to offer another choice. One meal — or even a series of meals — won't make or break the nutritional value of your child's diet.

- ✔ **Keep trying.** If your child doesn't like a particularly nutritious food, such as broccoli or oranges, offer the choice again at a later meal without pressuring your child to taste it. It may require several attempts to convince your child to try a new food.

Don't forget, too, that what *you* eat is important as well. Your child will notice and be influenced by what he sees you eat. See the earlier section "Modeling healthy choices" for more information on leading by example.

Limiting the junk

When you choose for your children to go dairy-free, taking steps to ensure that you replace the dairy you're ditching with foods that are comparable — and not worse than — the foods they're replacing is important. In other words, if your child stops drinking cow's milk, don't let soft drinks or highly sugared juices stand in for the beverage with meals.

Your child can eat only so much over the course of a day. Any time that your child consumes junk over nutrient-dense foods, she lessens the nutritional value of her diet. She decreases the likelihood that she'll get what she needs and increases the likelihood that she'll get too much of what she doesn't need. For example, when junk displaces nutritious foods, she tends to eat a lower amount of dietary fiber, vitamins, and minerals and a higher amount of saturated fat, trans fat, added sugars, and sodium.

If your child has access to junk foods regularly, she's more likely to become conditioned to eating junk and carry that habit into adulthood. Most junk foods come in the form of snacks — cakes, cookies, snack crackers, chips, candy, and other processed snacks foods. Instead of these, offer your child healthier snack options. (See the nearby sidebar "Healthful dairy-free snacks for children" for suggestions.)

Keep healthful, dairy-free snack options in plain sight where they're easy to grab when a snack attack strikes. A large bowl of colorful, ready-to-eat fresh fruit on the kitchen counter or table is a good idea. Keep several types of fruit on hand at any given time, including seasonal fruits such as berries, peaches, and melons.

Young children may need an adult or older child to help peel and cut some fruits such as oranges or apples. Be aware, too, that whole grapes may pose a choking hazard and shouldn't be given to children under 4 years of age.

Healthful dairy-free snacks for children

Make sure that snacks are nutrient dense. Good choices for children include the following:

- Celery with peanut butter*
- Whole-grain cereal with nondairy milk
- Fresh fruit
- Frozen fruit bars
- Muffins made with nondairy milk
- Pita points with hummus
- Fat-free microwave popcorn or popcorn made at home with vegetable oil*
- Sandwich half made with whole-grain bread

- Smoothies made with nondairy milk and fresh fruit
- Soup cups
- Tortilla chips with black bean dip
- Veggies with nondairy dressing or hummus*
- Whole-grain bagels with nondairy cream cheese
- Whole-grain toast with nondairy margarine and jelly

* Note that these foods shouldn't be given to children under 4 years of age because they pose a choking risk.

Sidestepping dairy at school

One of the mainstays of the school lunch tray is that squatty half-pint carton of cow's milk. Dairy products have always figured prominently in the national school meals program. In fact, in the National School Lunch Program — our nation's program for providing children with a hot, nutritious meal each day at school — it has long been a rule that for the meal to qualify for federal support, it has to include a serving of fluid cow's milk. Even if the child doesn't want it or doesn't drink it, that carton of milk has to be on the student's tray for the school to get federal credit for the meal.

In addition to cow's milk, the nation's surplus cheese has traditionally been funneled into the program, encouraging its use in many of the dishes served to our kids. Like milk, cheese is a government commodity that schools can get at a much-reduced price, increasing the incentive of schools to find a way to incorporate the food into lunch menus.

Dairy in school meals has been one of the factors responsible for the difficulty schools have had in reducing the saturated fat content of meals. Most school lunches still don't meet federal standards — the Dietary Guidelines for Americans — for limiting the amount of saturated fat in meals.

I mention it earlier in this book, but it bears repeating: Two-thirds of the fat in dairy products is artery-clogging saturated fat. That's a substance children and adults alike consume in excess, raising their risk for coronary artery disease and blood fat abnormalities, even in young people.

So what are your options if you want or need (for allergy or intolerance purposes) your child to avoid dairy products at school? Here are a few ideas:

✔ **Get a doctor's order.** Schools can give your child a nondairy alternative to cow's milk, such as fortified soymilk or rice milk, if his doctor writes a note attesting that he needs it for health reasons, such as an allergy or intolerance to cow's milk.

✔ **Coach your child.** Work with your child to help him pick and choose appropriately among the items offered on the menu each day. Review the menu with your child before he leaves for school each day, discuss the options, and help him determine what he may choose.

✔ **Work with school personnel.** Explain your child's food preferences or requirements to the school food service director and determine how the school may be able to accommodate and help your child.

✔ **Take it from home.** If it's too difficult for your child to consistently get what he needs from the school's lunch program, pack a lunch to send with him.

Avoiding dairy at parties, play dates, and other events

Social situations can be particularly challenging for kids on special diets. For a child who's living dairy-free, parties, play dates, school trips, holiday events, and other occasions with her friends often include food. When they do, staying dairy-free may mean that the child has to pass up the ice cream sundaes, the ice cream scoops on cake, and the slices of pizza.

REMEMBER Your child may find it unfair that she has to stay dairy-free when these foods are served. The key is to plan ahead for these situations. Before the event, discuss the options she's likely to encounter and talk through the possible choices.

TIP In many cases, you may be able to come up with a simple solution to help your child feel like she's included in the fun. You may be able to speak with the event planner ahead of time — a parent, teacher, or other adult — and make arrangements to bring a nondairy option for your child to eat and others to try. For example, if your child attends a birthday party, you may arrange to send along a half gallon of her favorite nondairy ice cream. She can have a scoop on her own slice of cake and share the rest with her friends.

Teaching kids to spot the dairy

When you decide to go dairy-free with your children's diets, you want to make sure they don't mistakenly eat dairy products. The best way to do so is to educate your children about what dairy is and what it looks like (check out Chapter 5).

Talk to your child about food and include him in meal planning. Doing so is the best way to teach him how to make appropriate food choices for himself. Take your child with you when you go grocery shopping, and explain how to read food labels. Show him how to work with recipes, and let him help with preparing meals. As I describe throughout this chapter, empower your child to take charge of his own diet.

Getting the family involved in the switch to dairy-free

As a longtime soymilk drinker, my carton of soy-milk kept company in the refrigerator with my husband's half gallon of cow's milk when we moved into our first home together. My husband, however, was influenced by my example and soon made the switch as well.

Throughout the years, we kept cow's milk in the refrigerator for our school-aged children, but we found at times that soymilk was all we had on hand. Eventually, the kids made the switch as well. Kids like what they become accustomed to, and ours soon thought nothing of pouring soymilk over their morning cereal.

When my husband and son found they were allergic to soy, they switched to rice milk. For years, we kept both soymilk and rice milk in the house.

Today, our college-aged daughter keeps cartons of soymilk in her dorm room refrigerator. Soymilk doesn't spoil as quickly as cow's milk, she says. Our younger son sometimes asks for cow's milk, and when he does, I buy a half gallon of the nonfat, organic variety. Dairy foods, while not entirely gone from our diets, are now nothing more than occasional ingredients.

Chapter 19

Aging Healthfully: Dairy-Free Diets for Older Adults

In This Chapter

▶ Recognizing your nutrition needs as a dairy-free older adult

▶ Maintaining healthy bones through your diet and lifestyle

*A*s the years go by, most people begin to realize that nothing stays the same forever. That's true of politics, other people, your backyard, and your body. As you get older, your hair turns grey, you lose muscle mass, and you need fewer calories each day to maintain your ideal weight. These changes aren't bad or good; they're just the realities of getting older.

But as you age, it's important to understand how the changes in the way your body works affect your nutritional needs, especially when you incorporate a dairy-free lifestyle. In other words, you need to know how to use your diet to support the best health possible for as long as possible. This chapter clears up everything for you.

Unfortunately scientists don't have all the answers yet. The science of *gerontology,* the study of normal aging, is still in its infancy. But scientists are gaining many insights into the patterns of change that many people experience as they age. You may take some of those changes for granted as being a normal part of aging, but they often occur at different times for different people.

Some people never develop certain conditions, such as osteoporosis. These differences among people may be due to genetic variations, but they're also almost certainly a result of lifestyle factors, including diet. You can stay healthy and feel better longer by eating the best diet possible.

In this chapter, I explain the changes you can expect to experience as you age, and how your dairy-free food choices can help you meet your body's changing needs.

Going Dairy-Free Later in Life

You needed milk when you were a baby, but by the time you were walking and talking, your days of feeding from the milk bottle or breast were over. You didn't need milk again as a young adult or in middle age. And contrary to what people say about going backward and becoming dependent again when you're old, no one will ever go back to needing a bottle or pacifier when he or she is 80. Living dairy-free for the rest of your life is okay.

Dairy products don't have any special nutrients that you can't get from other foods. As a matter of fact, you actually can gain some health advantages by eating a dairy-free diet throughout adulthood (check out Chapters 1 and 2 for more details).

Still, you need to understand how your nutrient needs change as you age and how to best meet those needs on a dairy-free diet. Being aware of your needs is especially important given the context in which most people live — in a world where dining with dairy is the norm. You're bound to hear questions and comments about your diet from people who aren't familiar with any other way of living. In this section, I give you an overview of your nutritional needs as you age.

Knowing how nutrient needs change over time

You may not realize that older adults have received relatively little attention from nutrition researchers over the years. In fact, information about the nutritional needs of people 50 and younger is more prevalent than for people older than 50.

As a result, scientists don't know as much about how aging affects your body's ability to digest, absorb, and retain nutrients. In the absence of research that specifically targets older adults, scientists extrapolate the needs of older adults from recommendations for younger people. One thing scientists do know, however, is that your metabolism declines over time. You need fewer calories to maintain the same body weight when you're 70 as compared to when you were 30.

Of course, your level of physical activity must stay the same. If you become less active as you age, you likely need even *fewer* calories to maintain the same weight. What's even more important to know is that as your calorie needs decline, it becomes even more critical that the foods you eat provide plenty of nutrients. In other words, you still have to get all the nutrients your body needs, but you have to get them from fewer foods. Think of it this way: Your calorie budget is smaller.

As a result, you have much less room in your diet for *empty-calorie foods* — junk foods, soft drinks, alcohol, and other low-nutrition foods and beverages — than when you were younger. Empty-calorie foods are nutritional freeloaders. They take up space and displace other more nutritious foods that you need in your diet. (Check out the later sidebar, "Jettisoning the junk" for ways to lower your intake of empty-calorie foods.)

Eyeing nutrients that need your attention

Although researchers don't know a lot about how nutrient needs change over time, they do have some information. In particular, some evidence shows that aging may diminish your body's ability to absorb certain nutrients. This diminished nutrient absorption happens because of changes in your *physiology* (the way your body functions, including the cells, tissues, and organs in your body) that make absorption less efficient. The following sections identify some nutrients in particular that you need as you age.

Your diet needs to be as nutrient-dense as possible to help ensure you get enough of what you need. The more junk you eat, the less room there is in your diet for the good stuff!

Vitamin B12

Vitamin B12 is a nutrient you need for the proper functioning of enzymes that help to regulate the metabolism of amino acids and fatty acids. Recommended dietary intakes of vitamin B12 are small — only 2.4 micrograms per day — but you need to pay special attention to this nutrient as you age.

As you get older, your body may produce less stomach acid, and stomach acids help the body absorb vitamin B12. Vitamin B12 is only found in animal products, such as meats, poultry, fish, eggs, milk, and other dairy products. So when you go dairy-free, you remove a common source of vitamin B12 from your diet.

Older adults are encouraged to eat foods that are fortified with vitamin B12, such as many cold cereals, or to regularly take a vitamin B12 supplement. This advice is especially important for vegetarians, vegans, or those who are limiting their intake of animal products, including dairy products.

A vitamin B12 deficiency can cause a form of anemia and a breakdown in the nerves in your hands, feet, legs, spinal cord, and brain. Symptoms of deficiency may include numbness, tingling, or burning in your feet or hands, and the effects may be irreversible.

Jettisoning the junk

As you age, especially beyond age 50, you need to limit your intake of junk foods. This advice is especially true if you're living a dairy-free lifestyle. As people age, they often include as many junk foods in their diet as they did when they were younger — and some eat even more of them. Why? Consider the following:

✔ The sense of taste or taste acuity often diminishes as people age, making very sweet or salty foods more flavorful and appealing.

✔ Many of those foods also take little time to prepare. Chips and crackers, cookies, commercially baked pies and cakes, and other desserts and processed snack foods are quick and convenient to eat and taste good.

The challenge, then, is to come up with ideas for alternatives to keep on hand that are nutritious and can take the place of less nutrient-dense snacks and treats. Swapping an apple for a chocolate chip cookie may not be easy, but doing so can improve the quality of your diet. Some ideas for handy, healthful dairy-free snacks and treats include

✔ Apple crumble (homemade with minimal sugar)

✔ Baked apple with a small scoop of nondairy ice cream

✔ Baked pita chips with hummus (you can find a hummus recipe in Chapter 12)

✔ Bowl of rice pudding made with almond milk or soymilk

✔ Bran muffin or other whole-grain muffin

✔ Flavored soy yogurt

✔ Fresh seasonal fruit cut into a fruit salad (see Chapter 9 for a recipe)

✔ Fresh strawberries topped with plain soy yogurt

✔ Frozen banana or grapes

✔ Vanilla soy yogurt with a dollop of fruit preserves

✔ Fruit smoothie made with nondairy milk (see Chapter 14 for some recipes)

✔ Homemade oatmeal cookie with fortified soymilk

✔ Low-fat or air-popped popcorn

✔ Toasted cinnamon and raisin bagel with trans-fat-free margarine

✔ Tortilla chips with salsa or black bean dip

✔ Whole-grain cold cereal with fortified almond milk

✔ Whole-wheat toast with trans-fat-free margarine and jam

You also can incorporate some strategies for keeping the junkiest foods to a minimum in your diet. Here are a few tips:

✔ **Put them away.** If you have packaged cookies, chips, and other snack foods around the house, keep them put away in the pantry or cupboard. If they're out of sight, you won't be reminded of them as often. Or, better yet, don't keep them in the house at all. If they aren't there, you can't eat them.

✔ **Go out instead of bringing them in.** If you have a hankering for a treat — a slice of pie or cake — go out and enjoy a serving at a restaurant. It's better than having a whole pie or cake at home, where one piece may lead to two — or more.

✔ **Display something better.** Keep a big, colorful bowl of seasonal fruit on your kitchen counter, or have a large bowl of fresh fruit salad waiting on the top shelf of your refrigerator. These treats can be constant reminders of your healthful eating habits when you're looking for a snack.

✔ **Minimize your intake of processed foods, and instead choose whole foods.** Doing so means eating a whole banana instead of a banana-flavored muffin, and eating a bowl of hot, cooked oatmeal instead of an oatmeal granola bar. I cover the essentials about nutrients you need and how to get them with a dairy-free diet in Chapter 4. I also discuss the pros and cons of relying on vitamin and mineral supplements to get what you need.

Calcium and vitamin D

Recommended intakes of calcium and vitamin D increase with age. If you don't drink cow's milk, which is concentrated in calcium and fortified with vitamin D, you must make sure you're getting enough of those nutrients from other sources — especially women, who are susceptible to *osteoporosis,* a calcium-deficiency disorder that can cause brittle, easily broken bones. (I discuss bone health more in the later section "Eating for Bone Health.")

Here's how to get the appropriate amounts of calcium and vitamin D:

✔ Get controlled amounts of sunlight exposure so your body can manufacture the vitamin D you need.

✔ Drink calcium- and vitamin D–fortified soymilk, rice milk, almond milk, or other forms of nondairy, fortified milk.

✔ Get plenty of calcium from rich food sources, such as beans, greens, sesame seeds, figs, and blackstrap molasses, or from foods fortified with calcium. Or you can take a calcium supplement. (I discuss calcium and vitamin D in detail in Chapter 4, including good food sources and how to get enough on a diet that's free of dairy products.)

Taking in whole foods to meet your vitamin and mineral needs

Because you need less food as you get older, and because your need for certain nutrients increases, it's as important as ever to eat well when you're making the transition to a dairy-free diet. The best way to do that is to focus on eating *whole foods* — those that are as close to their natural state as possible — to ensure that you're getting your required amounts of vitamins and minerals.

When starting your dairy-free diet, you want to strive to get what you need from food, not supplements. Food is the most foolproof source of essential nutrients, including those that haven't yet been identified by science and those that aren't packaged in a pill or tablet. Save supplements for times when you want a stop-gap measure or extra insurance if you think you may not be eating right. Just keep in mind that supplements don't replace an overall healthful diet.

Eating for Bone Health

Maintaining healthy bones as you age is very important. Getting enough of the right nutrients — including the calcium and vitamin D found in milk and other dairy products — is only one aspect of eating for bone health. If you don't eat dairy products (and even if you do), it's important to understand all the ways in which your lifestyle choices affect your bone health.

If you have poor bone health, you're at risk of developing osteoporosis, a major health threat for millions of older adults, most of them women. *Osteoporosis* is a condition characterized by bones that become porous and brittle. They may break easily, sometimes simply by sneezing too hard or falling down. For older adults, hip fractures caused by osteoporosis can be life-threatening and can cause loss of independence or a need to live in a nursing home or assisted living facility.

In this section, I explain what you need to know to keep your bones as healthy as possible as you get older.

Ensuring you get what you need

Getting plenty of calcium and vitamin D is one way to help protect your bone health. In Chapter 4, I provide detailed information about food sources of calcium, vitamin D–fortified foods, and the basics of how your body makes vitamin D from exposure to sunlight. I also provide a list of calcium-rich meals you may enjoy.

In this section, I focus on foods that are rich in calcium and vitamin D and also quick and convenient to buy or prepare. They're also in keeping with the overall nutritional goals for older adults — as nutrient-dense as possible while still satisfying aging taste buds!

For bone health, try the following meal suggestions that are high in calcium and vitamin D:

✔ **Canned black bean soup topped with chopped onions and grated nondairy cheddar-style cheese:** Add a mixed greens salad (using pre-washed, packaged salad greens is convenient) and a big chunk of hearty, whole-grain bread. Compare brands and shop for soups that contain the least amount of sodium. Natural foods stores carry the widest variety of soups with lower levels of sodium.

✔ **Hot oatmeal with slivered almonds, dried cranberries, cinnamon, and a teaspoon of brown sugar:** Serve it with fortified soymilk or almond milk and a glass of calcium-fortified orange juice. Use quick-cooking oats if you want to be quick. Leftovers are good reheated.

✔ **Baked potato topped with steamed, chopped broccoli (frozen is quicker to prepare than fresh), salsa, grated nondairy cheddar-style cheese, and a dollop of plain, nonfat soy yogurt:** Add a baby spinach salad (use prewashed, packaged spinach greens to save time) with sliced, fresh strawberries. Have half of a fresh orange for dessert.

✔ **Premade hummus on toasted pita bread points, bell pepper, and carrot sticks and a glass of calcium-fortified orange juice:** You can buy hummus in supermarkets or warehouse stores. If you have time to make your own, check out Chapter 12 for a recipe.

✔ **Quesadilla made with a whole-wheat flour tortilla, nondairy cheddar-style cheese, and chopped spinach (heat frozen spinach in the microwave oven):** Serve with salsa, avocado slices, a few black olives, and a scoop of plain, nonfat soy yogurt. For dessert, try a dish of rice pudding made with fortified soymilk and sprinkled with cinnamon and chopped walnuts.

Preventing calcium loss

Certain diet and lifestyle factors can diminish your body's ability to absorb and retain calcium in your bones. In Chapter 4, I discuss the general factors that can help you prevent calcium loss. All these factors are relevant to you as you age. However, a few of them merit special consideration for older adults. I explain them in the following sections.

Minimizing sodium in your diet

Older adults are notorious for spending less time cooking meals from scratch. In part, that's because they often live alone or with only one other person. They have less incentive to spend time cooking big meals when so few people are at home to enjoy them. Many older adults also don't want to have large quantities of leftovers to use up. Eating the same dish for days can be boring!

As a result, many older adults rely on frozen entrees and other prepared foods, which tend to be higher in sodium than many homemade meals. Like high protein intakes, high sodium intakes cause your body to lose calcium (not to mention contribute to high blood pressure). So try your best to read labels and choose products that are lower in sodium.

After you change your taste threshold for salt, regular soups and other salty foods you once enjoyed will taste too salty. The following are good ways to minimize the sodium load of your meals:

- ✔ **Dilute the sodium.** Include plenty of fresh fruits and vegetables in your diet to help dilute or offset other foods that may be higher in sodium. In other words, by eating more fruits and vegetables, which are naturally low in sodium, you can help balance out your nutrient intake. Aim to eat at least a couple of pieces of fresh fruit every day. Adding a fresh greens salad to meals also is a good idea.

- ✔ **Shop for low-sodium products.** Many grocery stores carry reduced-sodium products, such as canned tomatoes, canned soups, and condiments with less sodium than their traditional counterparts. Many canned vegetable brands now also carry products that have no added salt or are lower in sodium than the original products. Even if you add some salt while cooking, you're still getting much less sodium than you would if you bought the original salted variety.

- ✔ **Shake the salt habit.** Remove the saltshaker from your kitchen table, and get out of the habit of adding salt to the water when you cook hot cereal, pasta, or rice.

- ✔ **Season with alternatives.** Use sodium-free herb and spice blends to flavor foods. If you use bouillon, buy sodium-free or reduced-sodium brands.

A good way to add a dash of flavor to foods without adding sodium is to shake a few shots of cayenne pepper, red pepper flakes, vinegar, or low-sodium hot sauce onto foods.

Exercising regularly

You become less active as you age, but staying physically active as much as possible is important whether you go completely dairy-free or not. Why? Check out these reasons:

- ✔ **Weight-bearing exercise promotes calcium retention by your bones and helps to keep them strong.** Walking, hiking, skiing, playing volleyball, and other activities where you're active on your feet are all considered weight-bearing exercises. Take your healthcare provider's advice about the frequency and intensity of exercise that's right for you. However, generally speaking, moderate physical activities such as walking are appropriate for most people.

Aim for at least 2½ hours of moderate activity or 1¼ hours of vigorous-intensity aerobic activity each week. Include moderate to intense muscle-strengthening activities such as lifting light weights at least twice a week.

✔ **Physical activity is important because it helps keep your muscles strong.** Being strong and in shape, which includes having a good sense of balance and limber joints and muscles, makes you less likely to suffer falls. Fewer falls equals fewer broken bones.

✔ **Active people burn more calories, and the more calories you need, the more food you can eat.** The more food you eat, the more likely it is that you'll get all the nutrients you need to support good health. Now that's a good reason to get moving!

The U.S. government has issued physical activity guidelines for adults, including those over the age of 65. Read more detailed information online at www.health.gov/paguidelines/guidelines/chapter5.aspx.

Earlier recommendations for conserving your body's calcium stores also included advice to moderate your protein intake. For many years, nutritionists had warned that high-protein diets — typical for most Americans — increased the loss of calcium from bones. A more recent analysis of the research, though, suggests that this may not be a concern. I discuss this topic in more detail in Chapter 4.

Implementing strategies to maintain bone health

Eating right and being physically active can help you maintain healthy bones as you age. However, good intentions aren't always enough to ensure that a plan gets implemented. As I mention earlier in this chapter, many older people live alone or with only one other person, which can take some of the incentive out of cooking homemade meals. Likewise, if you exercise by yourself, staying motivated may be difficult.

To avoid these issues, think about ways to help support your efforts at living dairy-free as healthfully and as long as possible. Various strategies may work. Give some of these a try:

✔ **Exercise with a buddy or a group of buddies.** Having a social outlet can make physical activity much more enjoyable for many people. In fact, you may be helping others as you help yourself. So scout out your neighborhood, clubs, or other community groups for individuals who may want to participate in regular activities such as walking, working in a community garden, hiking, or playing tennis. Don't limit yourself to one activity. Get involved in more than one if you can find partners who would like to participate with you. After all, variety is the spice of life!

✔ **Organize potluck dinners.** Many people feel more like cooking — and eating — in social settings. So spread the work around and enjoy your collective efforts. Better yet, why not organize potlucks with a dairy-free theme, where everyone comes with their favorite dairy-free, calcium-rich dish?

✔ **Batch cook and freeze.** Part of the reason that older people don't enjoy cooking is that it's difficult to cook in small amounts for only one or two people. But if you take some time now and then to cook in batches, you can freeze part of what you make and then reheat it another day. You get the benefit of home-cooked meals (dairy-free and healthy), but you only have to eat enough for one meal.

✔ **Keep a food and exercise diary.** By keeping a written record of what you eat as well as how often and what kind of activity you engage in, you'll remain more aware of your lifestyle habits. Being aware of what you're eating and how often you're exercising can help keep you motivated and prevent you from lapsing on your healthy living.

Part V
The Part of Tens

The 5th Wave   By Rich Tennant

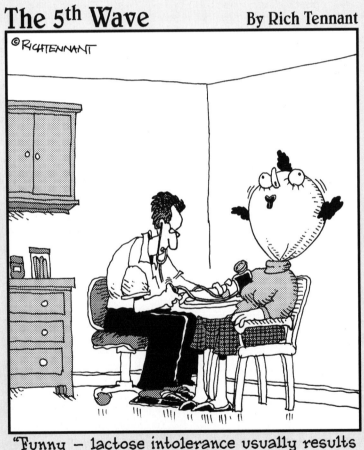

"Funny — lactose intolerance usually results in bloating of the stomach."

In this part . . .

To send you on your way, this book ends with five chapters designed to provide essential information about living a dairy-free lifestyle. All these chapters are in traditional *For Dummies* style: quick and to the point.

I start off with ten good reasons to go dairy-free, and then I follow that up with a summary of the best-tasting and most practical dairy-free products you'll find on the market. Next, I tick off a quick list of ten surprising places you may find dairy ingredients as well as ten ways to make going dairy-free easier on your wallet. Finally, I show you ten ways to get your kids involved with dairy-free eating.

Chapter 20

Ten Good Reasons to Dump Dairy

No biological evidence shows that your body requires you to drink or eat dairy products, so shake any concerns you may harbor about living dairy-free. Many good reasons support why everyone should consider reducing or eliminating their consumption of milk, cheese, yogurt, ice cream, sour cream, and other dairy foods.

I describe ten of these reasons in this chapter. One of these reasons may have been the one that initially compelled you to pick up this book. But after perusing all the other reasons to remove dairy products of your life, you may wonder why you didn't do it sooner. Collectively, the ideas I share may add weight to your decision to go dairy-free.

If you were undecided when you picked up this book, the information in this chapter should help to clinch your inclination to hop over to the dairy-free side of the fence. Read on, my friend. There are many compelling reasons to start living dairy-free. Which ones speak to you?

Cow's Milk Isn't Meant for Humans

Have you ever wondered why people drink milk from cows but not from dogs or pigs or elephants or moose? When you think about it, a cow's-milk habit is a little weird.

Human babies need milk from their human mothers. After they're weaned from breast milk, they don't need milk any more. Some people don't tolerate it beyond childhood, because their bodies can't fully digest it any more. So, in general, it's always best to stick with milk from your own species. After all, that's what Mother Nature intended.

Saturated Fat Hardens Arteries

Saturated fat is the key food ingredient responsible for making your body churn out the cholesterol that collects on and hardens your artery walls. Two-thirds of the fat in dairy products is saturated fat. Even so-called low-fat cheeses and low-fat milk are still high in saturated fat.

Hard, narrow arteries set you up for heart attacks and strokes. Those are big prices to pay for enjoying cheese on your broccoli and anything but nonfat milk with your cookies. The good news is that it doesn't have to be that way.

You can have all the foods you already love without the drawbacks of dairy. Nondairy alternatives to cheese, ice cream, milk, yogurt, and other dairy products contain little or no saturated fat and are kind to your arteries. You can read more about these alternatives in Chapter 6.

Lactose Is Difficult to Digest

Most of the world's adults can't fully digest *lactose,* the form of sugar found in cow's milk. That's because after infancy, many people's bodies gradually stop producing *lactase,* the enzyme needed to break down lactose into smaller sugars that the body can absorb and use for energy. The exception is people of Northern or Northwestern European descent, who often have a genetic variation that enables them to continue producing lactase into adulthood.

For everybody else, foods containing lactose may result in a range of unpleasant symptoms caused by malabsorption of the natural sugar in milk. Those symptoms may include gas, bloating, abdominal cramps, nausea, and diarrhea. Check out Chapter 3 for more on lactose intolerance.

Milk — and the lactose it contains — is baby food. Think of it this way: The fact that most adults can't digest it is Mother Nature's way of making them grow up.

Milk Contains No Fiber

Dietary fiber is your friend. It absorbs fluid and helps your stool mass stay large and soft, making it easy to pass and preventing problems with constipation and hemorrhoids. It also helps to slow the absorption of sugar from your bloodstream, evening out your blood-sugar level. It helps to lower your blood-cholesterol level as well.

You need lots of fiber from food — the more the better. So you should eat very few foods that don't contain at least a little bit of fiber. Dairy products, for instance, contain no fiber. Every time you eat dairy products, it means you're not eating something else. That "something else" can be an apple, a slice of whole-wheat bread, or a bowl of oatmeal, all of which supply health-supporting dietary fiber. Think of it in terms of the opportunity cost of eating dairy.

Milk Is Linked with Health Problems

The adult human body isn't meant to drink milk from a cow. In fact, defying your biology may have health consequences. In addition to lactose malabsorption and symptoms of lactose intolerance, some people are allergic to the proteins in milk. Symptoms of a milk allergy can be similar to those of lactose intolerance, and they may cause unpleasant health problems like gas, bloating, and diarrhea.

Researchers trying to find a cause (and a cure) for autism, a developmental disorder, have been testing the hypothesis that *casein,* a milk protein, may be linked to the disorder. More research is needed before that link can be confirmed, however.

Thinking more broadly, eating dairy products in anything more than low to moderate amounts risks depriving yourself of enough of the other foods you need each day to optimize your health. Think of it this way: A glass of skim milk — one of the lowest-calorie dairy products you can choose — still contains nearly 100 calories. A couple dollops of sour cream or a chunk of full-fat cheese may contain twice that number of calories. And when you fill up on these high-calorie foods, you aren't eating the nutritious veggies and whole-grain items that help you remain healthy.

Instead of eating these dairy products, you can trade the calories for hefty, filling portions of brown rice, spinach, black beans, or fresh orange wedges. All these foods contain much-needed nutrients and none of the excesses — saturated fat, trans fat, and sodium, for example — that are linked with higher rates of coronary artery disease, some forms of cancer, diabetes, and other chronic diseases and conditions.

Cows Heat Up the Earth

Cows are warming the planet, and thus playing a role in climate change. A 2006 landmark report called "Livestock's Long Shadow" by the Food and Agriculture Organization (FAO) of the World Health Organization noted that methane gases produced by cows raised for meat and milk account for 18 percent of all greenhouse gas emissions. Those gases threaten the existence of many species of animals around the world — including humans. So by going dairy-free, you're helping to preserve the natural balance of life on the planet. If people didn't eat so much meat or drink so much milk, farmers wouldn't have to raise so many gas-producing cows. You can read the FAO's report online at `ftp://ftp.fao.org/docrep/fao/010/A0701E/A0701E00.pdf`.

Dairy Farming Wastes Water

Look at a map of the world, and it looks like we live on a blue planet. It's difficult to imagine that having enough water could ever be a concern. However, most of the blue that you see on the map is salty seawater that humans can't drink or use to irrigate crops.

Aquifers that supply people with fresh drinking water and water used to irrigate crops lie deep beneath the earth's surface. Intensive animal farming practices like dairy farming place heavy reliance on fresh water supplies to raise the animals and grow the feed used to support them. So the threat posed by your dairy habit is the risk of dwindling supplies of fresh water.

Worse, however, is the fact that the pesticides, herbicides, and fertilizers used to grow feed for cows contaminate water supplies. The vast quantities of nitrogen-filled waste that cows produce are polluters as well. The waste finds its way into rivers, streams, lakes, and bays, contaminating those bodies of water and killing the creatures that live in them.

Dairy Farming Pollutes the Air

Animal agriculture, including the production of dairy products, requires intensive use of fossil fuels such as oil, coal, and natural gas to support the range of activities involved in the business.

For example, fuel is needed to transport feed to factory farms, to run farm machinery, to operate the facilities where animals are housed, and then to transport the final products to stores and manufacturers. Fossil fuels also are needed to produce the fertilizers used to grow animal feed.

Use of these fuels to support animal agriculture causes emissions of carbon dioxide, nitrous oxide, and methyl mercury, which pollute not only the air but the water and soil, too.

Dairy Farming Spoils the Soil and Eliminates Trees

Animal agriculture — including dairy farming — takes a toll on the land. Humanity's dependence on dairy foods and other animal products requires intensive use of the land for grazing animals and growing their food. This contributes to soil erosion from use of the land to grow feed for animals as well as from overgrazing of animals on the land. In Iowa, for example, half of the state's rich topsoil, which took thousands of years to create, has been lost in less than 200 years of farming.

And as more land is being devoted to grazing and growing crops to feed livestock, more forests are being cut down. This deforestation is a problem because forests act like the planet's lungs, trading carbon dioxide for oxygen and keeping the air healthy for humans. Protecting and conserving the soil and trees are vital tasks to protecting human health.

The FAO reports that livestock now occupy about one-third of the arable land in the world. It's bad now but it's getting worse. Dairy consumption is forecasted to more than double in the coming years. In fact, according to the FAO, milk production is expected to rise from 580 million tons in 2001 to 1,043 million tons in 2050.

Dairy Farming Is Unkind to Animals

Some people go dairy-free out of kindness. They feel compassion for the animals that are suffering in factory farms in order to satisfy humanity's milk habit. Most of the milk sold around the world comes from animals treated like milk machines. These animals are packed into confined quarters and valued for little more than their abilities to produce large amounts of milk.

These animals — who feel pleasure and pain just like you and me — are given hormones to make them produce the maximum amount of milk possible. This practice causes *mastitis,* an infection of the udder. The condition is treated with copious amounts of antibiotics, which contribute to worldwide problems with antibiotic resistance in humans.

As if that's not bad enough, cows that no longer produce enough milk are killed for their meat. And it's standard practice to take male calves born to dairy cows — who have to keep having calves in order to continue producing milk — and raise them in small confinement cages for their flesh. These calves are fed low-iron diets and kept in tight quarters so their flesh is soft and pale.

Knowing the full truth about the dairy industry makes it difficult for some people to continue eating dairy products. They choose to live dairy-free out of compassion for the animals and in keeping with their ethical standards.

Chapter 21

Ten Useful and Great-Tasting Dairy-Free Products

In This Chapter

▶ Experimenting with tasty nondairy substitutes

▶ Exploring the available alternatives

*E*liminating dairy products from your diet is much easier with the wide range of good-tasting, versatile dairy-free products on the market today. Name a dairy product, and I can show you a great nondairy alternative. The added bonus is that, nutritionally, you're likely to come out ahead, because these products are generally rich in vitamins and minerals but low in or free of artery-clogging saturated fat.

In this chapter, I include a description of ten of my favorite nondairy products. I buy these products on a regular basis because they taste so good and work so well in a variety of recipes. As you move toward a dairy-free lifestyle, consider giving these products a try. I list them in order of their star status in my book. Judge them for yourself.

You can find the biggest selection of nondairy products at natural foods stores, but many neighborhood supermarkets also are beginning to carry them, too. I talk more about removing dairy from your kitchen by using non-dairy alternatives in Chapter 6.

Vanilla Soymilk

Like a light, creamy milkshake, vanilla soymilk is a treat. It has a mild, beany flavor that fans say they become accustomed to quickly. Vanilla flavoring lends a slightly sweet taste to this delicious and nutritious beverage. Fortified soymilk is the most similar of the nondairy milks in nutritional value to cow's milk. It's a healthful, tasty, versatile beverage you can enjoy in many ways.

For example, you can drink vanilla soymilk straight from the carton with a handful of your favorite cookies. You also can pour it over your cereal in the morning, or use it to make puddings, custards, and smoothies. You can bake with it as well. You can use vanilla soymilk cup for cup in any recipe that calls for milk. My favorite brand is Silk, but many private-label and store-brand varieties also are quite good.

Almond Milk

Are you allergic to soy? If so, almond milk may be your beverage of choice (that is as long as you're not allergic to nuts). If you're allergic to soy *and* nuts, check out the next section for another alternative. Like soymilk, almond milk has a light, creamy consistency and a mild, pleasing flavor. It also comes in a range of flavors. The most popular — and practical — flavors include plain and vanilla.

Keep the plain variety of almond milk on hand to use in savory recipes, such as creamed potatoes and cream soups. (Chapter 10 provides a recipe for Creamed Potatoes with Brown Gravy.) You can use vanilla-flavored almond milk in everything else — on your cereal in the morning, with a slice of chocolate cake, in baked goods, and even in your coffee.

Almond milk — like other forms of nondairy milk — is sold in the refrigerator case in half-gallon cartons and on grocery store shelves in aseptic, shelf-stable containers. I like Almond Breeze by Blue Diamond Growers, but several other good products also are available.

Rice Milk

Rice milk is the third runner-up among nondairy beverages on my list; however, it's one of the most popular and widely available nondairy beverages on the market today.

In part, rice milk's popularity is due to the fact that it has such a mild flavor. It's also thinner in consistency than soymilk or almond milk, and its clean, white color makes it look more like cow's milk, too. If you're allergic to soy and want an alternative to almond milk, rice milk is an excellent choice.

Rice milk is sold refrigerated in half-gallon containers as well as on the shelf in aseptic, shelf-stable cartons. Rice Dream is a popular brand, and there are many others, including private-label varieties.

Soy Coffee Creamer

Do you need to put something creamy in your coffee in the morning? Even though you're living dairy-free, you still have some choices. Chief among them is a delicious product that's available in most supermarkets and in all natural foods stores: soy coffee creamer. It's available in plain, hazelnut, French vanilla, and other flavors. It's sold in pint and quart containers, and it keeps for several weeks in the refrigerator. Silk and Trader Joe's make good products, and others are available as well.

 Although it's great in coffee, some people also like to use soy coffee creamer in place of milk to make nondairy ice cream. It's thicker and creamier in consistency compared to soymilk. The plain variety also is useful in making cream sauces and cream soups.

Soy Yogurt

Soy yogurt is an all-around nondairy winner and a great way to start any day. It's available in plain and flavored varieties. Some flavored varieties include lemon, lime, and vanilla. You also can find varieties that contain fruit. Just like yogurt made with cow's milk, most soy yogurts contain active cultures. Popular brands include, among others, Silk and WholeSoy & Co.

Soy yogurt is creamy and thick and can be enjoyed in all the same ways that you may have eaten dairy yogurt. For example, use plain soy yogurt as a substitute for sour cream on a baked potato or burrito, or use it to make dips and dressings. Use flavored or fruited varieties to make smoothies, to stir into a bowl of granola, or to add to a fruit salad as a rich, flavorful topping.

Nondairy Ice Cream

Some days, you just need a dish of ice cream. When you do, try any of a number of nondairy frozen dessert products on the market and widely available in natural foods stores. These products are made from a variety of ingredients, including soymilk, tofu, rice milk, and other nondairy ingredients. They're available in flavors similar to conventional ice cream, including vanilla, strawberry, chocolate, chocolate chip, mint chocolate chip, and others.

Use these products to make milkshakes, sundaes, ice cream pies, and double-scoop cones. Popular brands include Rice Dream and So Delicious. Many brands are on the market, and they all taste a little different. Experiment to find those you like the best.

Also try your hand at making your own nondairy ice cream at home. It's quick and easy (and fun on a summer day!). I include several recipes in Chapter 14.

Nondairy Cheese

Years ago I would have said, "No way!" to nondairy cheese. However, today nondairy cheeses have improved flavor and texture, and they melt more easily when they're heated. They may be made with a variety of ingredients, such as soy, rice, oats, nuts, and other ingredients, which help give the cheese a solid, cheese-like texture.

Soy cheese has the best melt-ability of all the nondairy varieties of cheese, and it works particularly well in recipes such as macaroni and cheese where the quality of the dish depends on the cheese melting into a smooth, creamy cheese sauce. If you're hankering for a creamy bowl of mac 'n' cheese, head to Chapter 10 for a recipe.

Most soy cheeses do contain *casein,* a milk byproduct. If you're particularly sensitive to this milk protein, or you want to avoid all animal products for other reasons, read the ingredient label to be sure the soy cheese you buy is casein-free. People who are lactose intolerant, though, may be able to eat soy cheese without difficulties.

Nondairy cheeses are available in many varieties, including cheddar, Swiss, mozzarella, pepper jack, American, and others. Vegi-Kaas (which contains casein), VeganRella, and Soymage are examples of some nondairy cheese brands. As always, other brands are available, including private-label varieties.

Dairy-Free Margarine

Do you need something to spread on your toast at breakfast or on your roll during dinner? If so, dairy-free margarine is a great option. The consistency and flavor of these alternatives are quite good. In fact, you probably won't notice much, if any, difference between these dairy-free products and other varieties of margarine. Dairy-free margarine also melts well.

I use nondairy, trans-fat-free margarine and love it. In addition to being dairy-free, these products are better for your health than butter or margarine that's made with partially hydrogenated oils because they're low in saturated fat and free of artery-clogging trans fats. Among many others, you can try Fleishmann's Light Margarine, Smart Balance Light, and Earth Balance. Experiment to see which ones you like best.

Nondairy Cream Cheese

If you love bagels, you probably love big smears of cream cheese on them. Face it: Jelly on a bagel just doesn't cut it. The good news is that nondairy cream cheese products work as a great replacement. They're creamy and spreadable, just like dairy cream cheese. They taste good, too. Find dairy-free cream cheese in the refrigerator case at any natural foods store. Brands you may try include Tofutti Better Than Cream Cheese, Soymage, and Follow Your Heart Vegan Gourmet Cream Cheese, among others.

You can use nondairy cream cheese in a wide variety of ways, including in recipes for cookies and brownies, and for dips and spreads. You can even use it to make old-fashioned cheesecake (though the cheesecake recipe I include in Chapter 14 uses tofu straight-up instead).

Nondairy Sour Cream

On a baked potato or blintz, nondairy sour cream delivers the same creamy goodness as its dairy-based cousin — with zero lactose and no artery-clogging saturated fat. You also can use nondairy sour cream on burritos and nachos and in recipes for dips and spreads.

Brands include Soymage, Tofutti Sour Supreme, Tofutti Better Than Sour Cream, and others. If you want to make a homemade sour cream alternative, check out Chapter 12, where I include a recipe for Tofu Sour Cream.

Chapter 22

Ten Hidden Sources of Dairy

Dairy products show up in the darnedest places. Okay, so you probably know that chocolate milk or the dried cheese in your favorite macaroni and cheese mix contains milk. However, you may not realize that dairy ingredients are added to other foods, too. Many dairy additions aren't obvious from the product name or picture on the package. Furthermore, manufacturers may change product formulas from time to time. A product that used to contain a dairy ingredient may no longer contain it, or a product you thought was dairy-free may have had a dairy ingredient added since you last looked.

If you suffer from lactose intolerance, don't be surprised and eat something that gives you gas and cramps. To avoid any possible discomfort, you can train yourself to pay attention to dairy details in product ingredient lists. This chapter includes ten hidden sources of dairy. See whether you can add to this list by putting your dairy detective skills to work at home or at the store.

Baby Formula

The only acceptable alternative to breast milk for human infants is synthetic formula devised to simulate human breast milk. Baby formulas come in the following two general varieties:

   ✔ **Milk-based formulas:** Not surprisingly, this type contains milk components such as casein or whey proteins. Milk usually is noted prominently on the front of the can.

   ✔ **Soy-based formulas:** These popular formulas are made with soy products and often are used when infants don't tolerate formulas made with cow's milk.

Other formulations are available by prescription for babies with special needs, such as formulas for premature infants, babies that can't digest fats, and babies with heart disease or other disorders or conditions. Some of them contain dairy and some don't, depending on the nature of the issue the formula is meant to address. Your pediatrician or pharmacist can advise you if your baby needs one of these formulations.

Baked Goods and Baking Mixes

Cakes, cookies, quick breads, and brownies may not look like they're drenched in milk or oozing with cheesy goodness. However, it's common for small amounts of these ingredients to be blended into the batter or mix. Sour cream, yogurt, buttermilk, and other dairy ingredients also may be used.

As always, read labels carefully. If you're buying baked goods from a bakery shop or farmer's market, an ingredient list may not be available for review. In that case, ask the baker whether you can see the recipe. If the recipe isn't available, just assume that some amount of dairy is included in the product.

If you have difficulty finding your favorite baked goods without dairy, try making your own and substituting nondairy milk in the recipe. Chapter 8 provides some tips for adapting traditional recipes to be dairy-free.

Breakfast Cereals

Even before you pour the milk over them, some breakfast cereals contain dairy ingredients. For example, Kellogg's Low Fat Granola with Raisins contains nonfat dry milk. Similarly, Post Trail Mix Crunch Cranberry Vanilla cereal contains whey. *Whey* is the liquid part of the milk that's left over after milk has been curdled to make cheese.

The required allergen disclaimer at the bottom of the ingredient list may show that a product "may contain" milk ingredients. No other dairy products may appear in the product's ingredient list, however. If you're very sensitive to dairy and need to avoid even traces of it, you should err on the safe side and avoid products bearing the "may contain" disclaimer.

Candy

Candy covers a lot of ground, including everything from gumdrops and candy canes to candy bars and Turkish delight. With all those different varieties of candy out there, you can assume that some of them are made with milk, cream, and other dairy ingredients.

A few examples of candies that contain dairy ingredients include caramel, milk chocolate, yogurt-covered raisins or nuts, and some types of dark chocolate. Tootsie Rolls, Snickers Bars, Reese's Peanut Butter Cups, and many other favorites all contain milk or other forms of dairy, too. Read labels or visit manufacturers' Web sites to find out whether your favorite is dairy-free.

Coffee Creamers

You probably already know that half-and-half, whipped cream, and heavy cream are all derived from milk. What you may not realize is that even some powdered and liquid coffee creamers also contain dairy ingredients. For example, Coffee-Mate Fat Free Original coffee creamer (both liquid and powder forms) contains sodium caseinate, which is made from the milk protein casein. International Delight coffee creamers also contain sodium caseinate. So be sure to check labels carefully.

If you want something to put into your black coffee, use soymilk, rice milk, or almond milk. You also can try a nondairy soy coffee creamer, available in plain, vanilla, and hazelnut flavors.

Creamy Liqueurs

You may not have given it much thought in the past, but some of those creamy liqueurs you enjoy in your coffee or hot chocolate (or on the rocks) may contain dairy products. For example, Bailey's Irish Cream is 50 percent fresh cream. Other examples made with cream include Saint Brendan's and Heather Cream, which are both whiskey-and-cream liqueurs like Bailey's. Crème de la Crème Maple Cream, a Canadian liqueur made with maple syrup and cream is another, and Dooley's is a toffee and cream liqueur.

If you suspect a liqueur may contain dairy but aren't sure, check online. Most manufacturers provide ingredient information on their Web sites.

High-Protein Drink Powders

High-protein shake and drink mixes — often sold to body builders as energy drinks or weight control aids — commonly contain whey protein, a milk byproduct. *Tip:* Don't waste your money on these products. They're expensive, and most people shouldn't pump themselves full of so much protein.

Instant Mashed Potatoes

When you make mashed potatoes from scratch, you probably use milk and butter to add flavor and creaminess. Food companies add powdered versions of the same ingredients when they formulate their box mix versions of this classic dish.

If you have instant mashed potatoes in your pantry, read the ingredient list on the package. Many contain one or more of the following: nonfat dry milk, whey powder, sodium caseinate, and butter powder. If you see these items, steer clear of instant potatoes and make your own. I include a recipe for Creamed Potatoes and Brown Gravy in Chapter 10.

Nutrition Bars

Whatever you call them — nutrition bars, energy bars, or sports bars — some of these fast snacks contain dairy ingredients. Examples include whey protein isolate or whey protein concentrate, cultured whey, nonfat milk, and natural flavors that contain milk. Manufacturers sometimes change the ingredients used in their products, so be sure to read ingredient labels to be sure of what you're buying.

I include regular ol' granola bars and even some cereal bars in this category as well, because they're similar. In general, they're all portable, dry snack bars made with a blend of cereal grains, sweeteners, nuts, or fruit — and of course milk products often sneak in. ***Note:*** Despite the hype, none of these types of bars are particularly good for you. In general, you're much better off nutritionally with a piece of fresh fruit instead of one of these processed food bars.

Sherbet

You may assume that fruity sherbet contains no dairy products. Wrong! It often contains milk or cream, which gives the frozen dessert a creamy texture similar to that of ice cream. In contrast, its cousin *sorbet* is an ice treat generally made with nothing but fruit juice, sugar, and, sometimes, alcohol. Nondairy varieties of sherbet and ice cream are available. Or, if you're feeling ambitious, you can make your own with my recipes in Chapter 14.

Chapter 23

Ten Ways to Make Dairy-Free Eating Easier on Your Wallet

In This Chapter

▶ Being creative about ways to save

▶ Shopping and cooking strategically

*N*o doubt about it: Living dairy-free can put your wallet on a diet, too. Specialty products such as nondairy milks and cheeses and dairy-free substitutes for cream cheese and yogurt often cost more than their dairy counterparts.

These products don't have to break your budget though. You can minimize added expenses for specialty products by shopping for and using these foods strategically. You can keep in mind several helpful steps to save you money and still allow you to enjoy some of the convenience foods that make it easier to live dairy-free.

In this chapter, I introduce you to ten smart ways to get the most from the many different kinds of specialty dairy-free products on the market. Use as many of these tips as possible. Collectively, they'll leave you with a fatter wallet — and maybe even a trimmer waistline.

Buy in Volume

Larger quantities often are a better value. That's because the more units a company can sell of the same item, the more efficiently it may be able to produce the product. As a result, the company can shave a little off the price, pass the savings on to you, and still make a profit. Everyone wins.

This bulk business strategy is the premise behind the savings at warehouse stores like Costco, BJ's, and Sam's Club. It's also the reason you often get a discount of as much as 10 percent when you buy caseloads of foods at other stores, too. For example, many natural foods stores and specialty stores offer a percentage off the price of a case of nondairy milk or a larger lot of another specialty item, such as a bushel of fruit or a full box of frozen burritos.

You won't necessarily see signs advertising case discounts, though. So be sure to ask store personnel or the store manager what the store's policy is on buying in volume.

Shop Around

Stores may vary widely in what they charge for the same product at any given time, so you want to take the time to comparison shop. To do so, watch ads and circulars for notices about special pricing that may be in effect for a period of time at a particular store. When you find good prices, you may want to stock up on items that will keep for several weeks or months in the freezer or pantry. If you save enough, it may even merit a special trip to the store just for that one item.

Larger stores that sell in volume often can offer lower prices. For example, large natural foods stores often sell nondairy milks and cheeses at substantially lower prices than you find at small health food stores or conventional supermarkets that don't stock a large selection of dairy-free products.

However, the specialty foods marketplace is changing rapidly, so don't assume anything. Check around to make sure you're getting the lowest price. More conventional supermarkets have started stocking soymilk, rice milk, and other nondairy milks, yogurts, and cheeses. As more people buy these products, you may see prices drop.

Make it a practice to stop in at different stores from time to time so you can keep tabs on which stores have the best prices for the products you like to buy. Making written notes of prices and quantities can be helpful; mental notes often get lost in the shuffle of daily life.

Share with a Friend or Family Member

What are friends and family for, if not for sharing with? For example, you may not need an entire case of almond milk this month, but it may be worth it to go in on it with someone. Splitting an order with a friend gives you the following advantages:

✔ **It saves you both money.** You can save money by buying in volume and splitting the product with a friend. When you run out, you can repeat the process to save and share again. Sharing works especially well when you buy perishables such as fresh fruit or refrigerated nondairy milks. It helps to ensure you'll reap the savings but also use the food before it spoils.

✔ **It saves you both space.** Why use up valuable refrigerator and pantry space by buying more than you need in the near future when you can split the order into a more manageable quantity with a friend or family member?

✔ **It minimizes the risk if you want to try something new.** For example, say that you've never tried a particular brand of mozzarella-style non-dairy cheese, and you're now ready to give it a whirl. Buy a block of the cheese and split it (along with the cost) with a friend. If you find you don't like it, you've each spent only half the amount you otherwise would have spent, and you may have wasted less. If you find you like the product, great! Buy it again — and this time in bulk — and then share and save some more.

Buy Generic

Generic, store brand, and private-label products typically cost less than their name-brand cousins. The same manufacturers that package brand-name items often make these no-name products. By buying the generic, you frequently get the same high-quality product for less than you'd pay for the leading brands. Examples of dairy-free generic, store-brand, or private-label products you're likely to see in stores include soymilk, rice milk, nondairy yogurt, and nondairy cream cheese.

Clip Coupons

A great way to save some money when eating a dairy-free diet is to use coupons. You can find coupons all around you. You just have to look. Consider the following options:

✔ You can find coupons in food-themed magazines, within in-store circulars, on store shelves, and on the products themselves (just peel and save). So be sure not to limit your search to the Wednesday food section of your local newspaper.

✔ Another good place to look for coupons is on manufacturer Web sites. It's becoming common for food companies to include on their Web sites not only recipes but coupons, too, which you can print and take with you to the store. Peruse sites for specific brands of soymilk, rice milk, almond milk, nondairy cheese, yogurt, and whipped toppings.

✔ You also can look on coupon Web sites. One good example is www.coupons.com. You can find hundreds of coupons for a wide range of products consolidated in one place.

Coupons can be a nice way to save money on staples or to get a discount on a product you'd like to try. Be smart, though, and don't let a coupon entice you into buying something you don't need or would ordinarily buy in its less expensive, store-brand form.

When clipping coupons, stay organized. Keep coupons together in one central spot — an envelope, basket, file folder, shelf, or even a favorite dish — where you know to look before you go to the store. Regularly look through your coupon stash and throw away any that have expired.

Make It Yourself

You may not have even considered making your own nondairy milk and cheese. Although few people are willing to go to the effort, making some nondairy foods isn't that difficult. For example, I include quick and easy recipes for Tofu Sour Cream and a maple-flavored, cream cheese-like spread in Chapter 12. And making your own nut milk is quite easy as well — check out Chapter 6 for details.

You also can use nondairy ingredients to make your own breads, entrees, desserts, and other foods that may cost more because they're nondairy specialty items. If you make these foods yourself, you can generate substantial savings over buying ready-made, dairy-free foods from the store. Check out the recipes I include in Part III of this book.

Eat at Home

You can eat more meals at home to save money. It's good advice for everybody, whether or not you're living dairy-free. The typical American spends 40 percent of his food budget on meals away from home. Think of all the money you can save and how much more control you can have over your meals if you ate at home instead of in restaurants.

Similarly, when you make your own dairy-free macaroni and cheese, lasagna, and casseroles instead of buying frozen, ready-to-heat products from natural foods stores, you save money. That's generally true even though some of the ingredients, such as nondairy cheese, are relatively expensive.

If you tend to eat out because you never know what to eat on any given day, try planning your meals and making a grocery list based on those meals. Because you'll always have meals on hand, you won't be as tempted to rely on eating out. See Chapter 7 for more information on shopping and stocking your dairy-free pantry.

Go Easy on the Cheese

All cheeses, dairy-based or not, are relatively expensive compared with other kitchen staples. Nondairy varieties of cheese tend to be even more expensive than dairy cheese.

 One way to trim some of the cost is to use cheese sparingly. For example, if you top a pizza with mozzarella-style nondairy cheese, sprinkle the grated cheese in a thin layer rather than applying it heavily. And use one slice of non-dairy cheese in a grilled sandwich, not two.

You can be frugal with other ingredients, too. Instead of serving a full bowl of expensive soy yogurt as a snack, serve a dish of fruit salad with a dollop of vanilla soy yogurt on top.

Throw Away Less

Be thrifty and try not to let things go to waste. For example, if you bought hemp milk and don't care for the flavor, use it up when you're making baked goods. Or try adding it to a fruit smoothie, where the flavor is disguised by sweet strawberries and kiwi.

If you have odd bits of nondairy cheese or small amounts of this and that, add them to other foods to use them up. For example, if you have small amounts of two or three different kinds of nondairy cheese, combine them and stir them into a casserole or use them on bean burritos.

Use Fewer Specialty Products

Products such as nondairy cheeses and milks, yogurt, sour cream, and others are convenient and can be fun to use. They taste good, too. Still, you don't need to eat these foods at every meal. You can use these specialty products less often and use alternate options that may be less expensive.

For example, sandwich fillings such as hummus, almond butter, and grilled veggies are healthful alternatives to processed cheese. And honey and jam are tasty, lower-calorie alternatives to nondairy cream cheese on a bagel. You also can use soymilk or another favorite nondairy beverage on your bowl of cereal in the morning, but then you can drink water as a beverage with other meals.

Chapter 24

Ten Ways to Make Dairy-Free Fun for Kids

In This Chapter

▶ Getting kids on board with dairy-free eating

▶ Creating enjoyment around the transition of living without dairy

There's a foolproof recipe for getting children to eat (and enjoy!) their dairy-free meals. The key ingredient? Fun! A hefty dose of fun can make any lifestyle change more comfortable to endure. And if your kids are happy, family meals will be a whole lot easier for everyone.

Pumping up the fun factor isn't difficult either. You just need to understand some simple strategies to get started. In this chapter, I share ten basic principles and tips for making dairy-free eating fun for the whole family. A good way to generate excitement about dairy-free foods is to kick things off by making a few all-time favorites. I share advice about this and other good ways to start.

Here's the most important point to remember from this chapter: Make sure you encourage your kids to dig in and be full participants in meal planning and preparation. Ensuring that your kids are included in these important food decisions can help prepare them to manage their diets as adults.

Get Their Input

Everybody has opinions about food, and kids are no exception. So make sure you find out their opinions. Look for opportunities to let your kids express their food preferences — what they like best, what they definitely don't like, and what they'd be game to try. Giving them a chance to weigh in on decisions about what you'll have for dinner is a good way to make them feel included. Doing so also encourages their buy-in on the transition to a dairy-free lifestyle. I discuss this tactic a bit more in Chapter 18.

You can even formalize your children's roles by creating a family food advisory board. Set aside regular times — once a month, for example — to sit down as a family and talk about what's working and what can be improved where meals are concerned. Use these meeting times to give family members an opportunity to raise issues of concern and to suggest potential solutions.

Take Them Shopping

Kids have more fun and a greater interest in meals when they have had a hand in creating them. Picking out and bringing home the ingredients you need to fix family meals is one way they can help and feel as though they're making a contribution in the transition to a dairy-free lifestyle.

To get them involved in the shopping, when you get to the store or farmer's market, give your kids an assignment. Young children can help pick out apples and oranges to put into your basket. You can give older children a short list and send them on missions to find what you need. For example, while you're perusing the produce aisle for fresh broccoli and kale, send your older child to the dairy case with instructions to pick out a carton of rice milk.

Be careful not to be too particular or critical of your child's choices at the start. Helping with simple grocery shopping tasks is a good way to build your child's sense of confidence and mastery of the job.

If he comes back with plain rice milk instead of vanilla, don't be overly concerned. Gently point out the difference and let him choose whether he wants to go back and make an exchange. Likewise, if the apple your child picks has a little bruise or other imperfection, let it slide. In the scheme of things, what's most important is that your child is learning — and having fun with it.

Teach Them to Cook

Like shopping, getting kids involved in the actual preparation of meals is a fun way to engage them in the art of living dairy-free. Kids of all ages can help in the kitchen and discover how to cook. Here's a list of what children may like to do during dinner preparation:

- **Younger children:** They can help with simple tasks, such as fetching ingredients, dumping ingredients into a pot that's not on the burner, or stirring ingredients in a mixing bowl.

- **Older children:** They can learn how to use measuring spoons and cups and how to follow a recipe. They also can learn how to turn on the oven and the proper way to stir foods on the stovetop (handles turned inward!) to reduce the risk of spills and burns.

Kids of all ages can benefit from learning kitchen safety tips and basic cooking techniques. Explain to them what you're doing as you cook and why. For example, when your child adds the grated, nondairy cheese to the bowl of pasta, you can explain how nondairy cheese melts best when it's mixed throughout the dish where other hot, moist ingredients can help it to melt. Besides getting children on board for living dairy-free, teaching them to cook builds confidence and self-reliance, which will help them in their adult lives.

Play the Taste Test Game

Experimenting with new dairy-free foods can be fun for you and your kids. Figure out what your children prefer and then use the results of the taste test to draft your next shopping list. In fact, you can turn tasting new foods into a game. To do so, set out samples of different kinds of nondairy milk — soy, rice, almond — and let the kids taste and evaluate them. Which ones are the creamiest and best-tasting? Ask whether they like vanilla or plain best.

Do the same with different styles of nondairy cheese — mozzarella, pepper jack, and cheddar, for example — and ask the kids to rate their favorites on a scale of 1 to 5, with 1 being best and 5 being worst.

Whip Up Some Smoothies

Everybody loves smoothies. They're tasty and easy to make. By whipping up nondairy smoothies, your kids can begin to enjoy a dairy-free diet. And everyone can be involved. Young kids can help by measuring and adding ingredients to the blender or food processor. Older kids can operate the appliances themselves.

Part of the fun of making smoothies is the opportunity to get crazy with creative concoctions. Let kids experiment with their own combinations of nondairy milk, fresh fruit, ice cubes, cocoa, decaffeinated coffee, and other ingredients.

As you and your children create new smoothie variations, make notes to remember which ingredients you added and how much of each. Have kids name their creations. I include some great smoothie recipes in Chapter 14 to get you started.

Make Dairy-Free Ice Cream

When kids realize that dairy ice cream is out when going dairy-free, they may be disappointed. So a great way to make the transition to a dairy-free lifestyle is to make your own dairy-free ice cream. Doing so is easy, and kids can still get to enjoy their favorite treat.

Here's the rundown on how to make your own homemade ice cream: Measure the short list of ingredients and dump them into an electric ice cream maker. Press the button and watch the liquid turn into a frosty, thick slurry (about 15 to 20 minutes). Wait a little longer, and the milkshake-like treat becomes scoopable excitement. I include more specific directions and some starter recipes in Chapter 14.

Play with Tofu

Tofu is a versatile and easy-to-use ingredient in many dairy-free dishes, so it's a good way to generate some kid-friendly fun. Let your kids become acquainted with tofu in the kitchen by trying it in their favorite meals.

Use tofu to make nondairy sour cream, which can top kid-friendly burritos, nachos, and baked potatoes. I include a recipe for it in Chapter 12. Also consider trying your hand at the Maple Nut Spread recipe — a delicious, nondairy cream cheese alternative — in the same chapter.

Finally, surprise everyone by using tofu to make a frozen, ice cream-like treat. I include recipes for Strawberry Tofu Ice Cream and Chocolate Tofu Ice Cream in Chapter 14.

Focus on Favorites

When making a change to a dairy-free lifestyle, you can show your kids that it's not that big of a deal by continuing to fix their favorite dishes. You can show them that they're favorites still look and taste the same even when you omit the dairy. Nondairy versions of many kid-pleasing foods are guaranteed to go over well.

Sure-fire choices include

- Multigrain Waffles (Chapter 9)
- Cream of Tomato Soup and Macaroni and Cheese (Chapter 10)

> ✔ Easy Vegetable Lasagna, Spaghetti with Marinara Sauce, Vegetable and Cheese Quesadillas, and Baked Seven-Layer Burritos (Chapter 11)
>
> ✔ Banana Bread, Cheeseless Pizza, and Mucho Nachos (Chapter 13)
>
> ✔ Strawberry Kiwi Smoothie, Favorite Chocolate Pudding, and different flavors of ice cream (Chapter 14)

Bake Cookies

Homemade cookies put a smile on everybody's face. Just because they're dairy-free doesn't mean they still can't be fun. To get started, get out the electric mixer and cookie sheets. Bake a couple of batches of your family's favorites. Use the guidance in Chapter 8 to replace the dairy products in your traditional, dairy-intensive recipes.

Then get ready to enjoy a handful of warm, freshly baked cookies with a tall, cool glass of vanilla soymilk. Your kids and their friends will think dairy-free is a great idea.

Have Fun Yourself

If you're having fun with your new dairy-free lifestyle, everyone around you will have more fun, too. It's part of the strategy of modeling the behavior — or attitude — you'd like others to adopt, particularly your children. Show them that it's not only easy to eat a dairy-free diet, but it's a jolly good time, too! Good times are contagious. The food is great, you get to have fun fiddling with new ingredients, and your kids can learn about good food along with you.

Index

• E •

Business/Accounting & Bookkeeping

Bookkeeping For Dummies
978-0-7645-9848-7

eBay Business
All-in-One For Dummies,
2nd Edition
978-0-470-38536-4

Job Interviews
For Dummies,
3rd Edition
978-0-470-17748-8

Resumes For Dummies,
5th Edition
978-0-470-08037-5

Stock Investing
For Dummies,
3rd Edition
978-0-470-40114-9

Successful Time
Management
For Dummies
978-0-470-29034-7

Computer Hardware

BlackBerry For Dummies,
3rd Edition
978-0-470-45762-7

Computers For Seniors
For Dummies
978-0-470-24055-7

iPhone For Dummies,
2nd Edition
978-0-470-42342-4

Laptops For Dummies,
3rd Edition
978-0-470-27759-1

Macs For Dummies,
10th Edition
978-0-470-27817-8

Cooking & Entertaining

Cooking Basics
For Dummies,
3rd Edition
978-0-7645-7206-7

Wine For Dummies,
4th Edition
978-0-470-04579-4

Diet & Nutrition

Dieting For Dummies,
2nd Edition
978-0-7645-4149-0

Nutrition For Dummies,
4th Edition
978-0-471-79868-2

Weight Training
For Dummies,
3rd Edition
978-0-471-76845-6

Digital Photography

Digital Photography
For Dummies,
6th Edition
978-0-470-25074-7

Photoshop Elements 7
For Dummies
978-0-470-39700-8

Gardening

Gardening Basics
For Dummies
978-0-470-03749-2

Organic Gardening
For Dummies,
2nd Edition
978-0-470-43067-5

Green/Sustainable

Green Building
& Remodeling
For Dummies
978-0-470-17559-0

Green Cleaning
For Dummies
978-0-470-39106-8

Green IT For Dummies
978-0-470-38688-0

Health

Diabetes For Dummies,
3rd Edition
978-0-470-27086-8

Food Allergies
For Dummies
978-0-470-09584-3

Living Gluten-Free
For Dummies
978-0-471-77383-2

Hobbies/General

Chess For Dummies,
2nd Edition
978-0-7645-8404-6

Drawing For Dummies
978-0-7645-5476-6

Knitting For Dummies,
2nd Edition
978-0-470-28747-7

Organizing For Dummies
978-0-7645-5300-4

SuDoku For Dummies
978-0-470-01892-7

Home Improvement

Energy Efficient Homes
For Dummies
978-0-470-37602-7

Home Theater
For Dummies,
3rd Edition
978-0-470-41189-6

Living the Country Lifestyle
All-in-One For Dummies
978-0-470-43061-3

Solar Power Your Home
For Dummies
978-0-470-17569-9

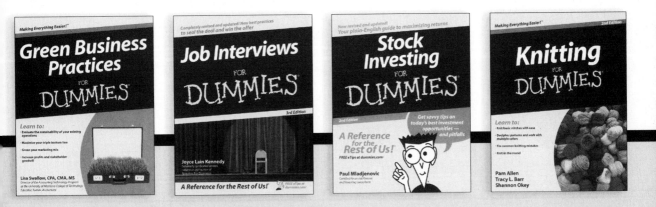

Internet
Blogging For Dummies,
2nd Edition
978-0-470-23017-6

eBay For Dummies,
6th Edition
978-0-470-49741-8

Facebook For Dummies
978-0-470-26273-3

Google Blogger
For Dummies
978-0-470-40742-4

Web Marketing
For Dummies,
2nd Edition
978-0-470-37181-7

WordPress For Dummies,
2nd Edition
978-0-470-40296-2

Language & Foreign Language
French For Dummies
978-0-7645-5193-2

Italian Phrases
For Dummies
978-0-7645-7203-6

Spanish For Dummies
978-0-7645-5194-9

Spanish For Dummies,
Audio Set
978-0-470-09585-0

Macintosh
Mac OS X Snow Leopard
For Dummies
978-0-470-43543-4

Math & Science
Algebra I For Dummies,
2nd Edition
978-0-470-55964-2

Biology For Dummies
978-0-7645-5326-4

Calculus For Dummies
978-0-7645-2498-1

Chemistry For Dummies
978-0-7645-5430-8

Microsoft Office
Excel 2007 For Dummies
978-0-470-03737-9

Office 2007 All-in-One
Desk Reference
For Dummies
978-0-471-78279-7

Music
Guitar For Dummies,
2nd Edition
978-0-7645-9904-0

iPod & iTunes
For Dummies,
6th Edition
978-0-470-39062-7

Piano Exercises
For Dummies
978-0-470-38765-8

Parenting & Education
Parenting For Dummies,
2nd Edition
978-0-7645-5418-6

Type 1 Diabetes
For Dummies
978-0-470-17811-9

Pets
Cats For Dummies,
2nd Edition
978-0-7645-5275-5

Dog Training For Dummies,
2nd Edition
978-0-7645-8418-3

Puppies For Dummies,
2nd Edition
978-0-470-03717-1

Religion & Inspiration
The Bible For Dummies
978-0-7645-5296-0

Catholicism For Dummies
978-0-7645-5391-2

Women in the Bible
For Dummies
978-0-7645-8475-6

Self-Help & Relationship
Anger Management
For Dummies
978-0-470-03715-7

Overcoming Anxiety
For Dummies
978-0-7645-5447-6

Sports
Baseball For Dummies,
3rd Edition
978-0-7645-7537-2

Basketball For Dummies,
2nd Edition
978-0-7645-5248-9

Golf For Dummies,
3rd Edition
978-0-471-76871-5

Web Development
Web Design All-in-One
For Dummies
978-0-470-41796-6

Windows Vista
Windows Vista
For Dummies
978-0-471-75421-3

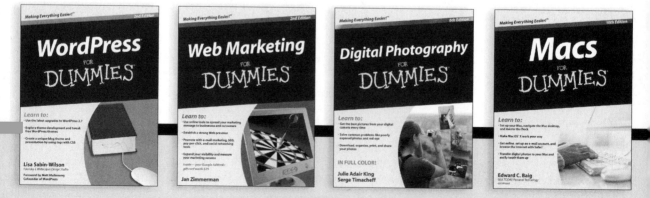

Available wherever books are sold. For more information or to order direct: U.S. customers visit www.dummies.com or call 1-877-762-2974.
U.K. customers visit www.wileyeurope.com or call (0) 1243 843291. Canadian customers visit www.wiley.ca or call 1-800-567-4797.

DUMMIES.COM®

How-to?
How Easy.

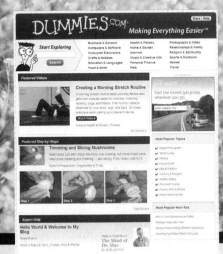

From hooking up a modem to cooking up a casserole, knitting a scarf to navigating an iPod, you can trust Dummies.com to show you how to get things done the easy way.

Visit us at Dummies.com

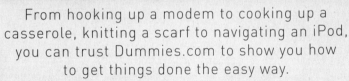

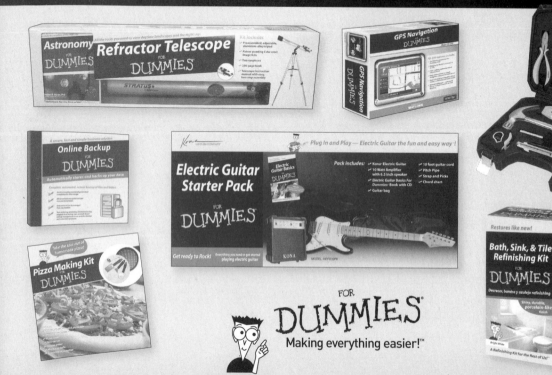